Entrapped

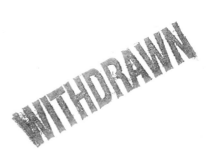

Entrapped

JUANITA MURPHY

ISBN-13: 9781516887859
ISBN-10: 1516887859

Author's Note

The central theme of these few shared experiences is that, in the process of traveling our life's journey, we may encounter obstacles that seem to be overwhelming. These obstacles vary in nature, severity, and longevity. Included in this limited treatise are some obstacles experienced by an individual who survived the devastating effects of a massive stroke; two caregivers' experiences caring for their loved ones following devastating strokes; and entrapments encountered by two individuals who had survived traumatic childhoods.

Interestingly, both survivors and caregivers described feelings and thoughts of being cornered or trapped, losing control, having no way out, lost independence, and worthlessness. One traumatic childhood survivor reported problems with extreme guilt. The other traumatic childhood survivor implied excessively aggressive behavior. Caregivers included feelings of extreme stress, isolation, hopelessness, abandonment, and exhaustion.

Both survivors and caregivers revealed some of their innermost feelings of anger, hate, anxiety, sadness, denial, frustration, rebellion, panic, agitation, fear, and depression. Problem drinking and thoughts of suicide were also disclosed. It is hoped that the revelation of these extremely negative feelings and thoughts, particularly anger and dislike of self and others, might be considered a natural reconstructive process and dealt with accordingly.

Each contributor was seeking an answer to the question, "Why has this happened?" The individuals had to consciously, or unconsciously, reshape their lives through enormous changes to escape from the entrapments that had been thrust upon them. Some turned to a higher power and pleaded for release from the bewildering and destructive forces that had invaded their lives. Others described how they had used inner strengths to develop coping strategies that were directed toward acceptance of the new reality.

Transitions out of the binding entrapments were arduous. Lifestyle adjustments rarely followed a planned course. Relationship problems often blocked the path to escape. Yet each contributor developed unfathomable strengths to face each day with a sense of fulfillment, albeit minimal on some days. Each shared story attests to the ability of human beings to deal with complex and overwhelming obstacles that thwart or obstruct our life's journey. Counseling or therapeutic groups might have lessened the anguish or sped up the recovery process. I hope that you may gain some insight into how to cope with similar obstacles that may be occurring in your life presently. Additionally, I trust that this limited sample of experiential sharing will be therapeutic for you, as it has been for each of us.

I know each of the contributors personally. I came up with the idea of "Entrapment", and shared my plans to write a book. Each person developed her/his story either in writing or by an interview with me. The stories began to add intent and integrity to the initial idea. It has been a tremendously fulfilling endeavor for me.

Some of the contributors elected to use pseudonym, and one opted to remain anonymous. Hopefully, this is not a distraction.

Table of Contents

One

Ten Years of Caregiving: A Love Story – Susan Brooks

This is a love story—an ordinary story that is being lived in my home and in many homes everywhere. Darryl's and my love story is only extraordinary in that it is ours. Many of the circumstances and details of our story are different, but I suspect there are also many similarities in other homes. When one person becomes the caregiver of a loved one, there is challenge and heartbreak as well as a thought-provoking, deepening process. This is the story of our ten-year journey through disease and caregiving, from the dramatic acute onset and on into chronic disease.

Darryl and I grew up in the quieter world of the mid-1940s and 50s. At an early age, I decided I wanted to be a nurse. I was drawn to medicine, or more accurately, to being a helper. I also thought nurses wore cute hats. After high school, I entered a nursing program, where the corollary values of patient care and sacrifice were drummed into our heads. The patient always comes first, first before your breakfast, lunch, or dinner, first before emptying your full bladder, just plain first. Darryl grew up an outdoorsman, not caring much about school, and wandering the woods, fishing and hunting. He joined the navy during his senior year of high school, and he shipped out shortly after graduation. He served as a corpsman (medic) in Vietnam, and on a submarine tender on the East Coast. After the military, he worked as a mental-health therapist on a psychiatric unit. We met at work, on a psychiatric unit where I was a newly hired nurse. He had been married for ten years and was divorced. I was widowed after twelve years of marriage. We each had two children when we married in 1980.

Over the years we raised the children, and we had an assortment of farm animals, including pigs, geese, goats, chickens, sheep, horses, and one burro. We always had a big garden, lots of wild blackberries, and a much-undisciplined yard. By 2005, the only animals that lived with us were two dogs and two goats. We had several grandchildren and celebrated being a family by getting together for Sunday dinner almost every week. Darryl had changed his career focus to hospital security, where he taught hospital staff about mental illness and behavior control. I had changed fields and had become a hospice nurse.

Enter the big change, or as I call it, Darryl's Big Event. On February 21, 2005, our worlds turned upside down. Darryl suffered a major heart attack and a stroke, and as a result of periodic cardiac arrest, an anoxic brain injury. These past ten years have been filled with growth, change, entrapment, and the struggle to find peace with it all. I have sat with my journals written over these years and am reminded of the sharp pain of loss, the struggles with resentment, the longing and loneliness, the fear, the months of soldiering through, and the continual search for meaning within all of this. I believe that this journey has given me growth and a serenity that I probably would not have found without such a major challenge.

I am the primary and sole caregiver for Darryl. Learning to ask for help, finding out what kind of help I need, making plans and letting go of them and starting over—all of this, and more, have been etched in the pages of my journals.

Saturday, February 26, 2005
To write about the events of this past week feels like it will make those events real. Real they are, however, in a nightmarish way that I am only beginning to comprehend. Darryl had a heart attack, and as a result, he has suffered several strokes. I do not know who will wake up

from this drug-induced coma. It is so hard to see him in that place of not being himself. And it is distressing that I don't know when or if he will return.

I transition between being numb, terrified, and grief-stricken. In the mornings, I feel optimistic, by afternoon I am devastated, and by bedtime, I am both of those and everything in between. The kids have circled the wagons, and the staff at the hospital has been wonderful. But it is still a catastrophic feeling. Some parts of me are in denial. Yesterday was a hard day because he looked more like himself but was still so unresponsive. We are in territory that has no recognizable landmarks since we are not familiar with life in the intensive care unit. I am angry that I was just feeling closer to this complicated man and now he is an enigma again. This marriage has been through a few incarnations, and I hope it will continue through a few more.

Monday, February 28, 2005
It has been one week. I feel like this must be what alcoholics and drug addicts feel when they "hit bottom." There is just nothing to do but surrender to the lack of control, to turn my life over to a higher power and pray.

My feelings are like a yoyo and seem pretty unreliable as a gauge of what is really happening. I woke up to a dream that Darryl sat up and looked around for a minute, even though he was still intubated.

Saturday, March 12, 2005
Either this is devastation, or it is an adventure. If I can manage to keep my thinking toward the adventure place, the challenging is not so overwhelming. Here we are, doing the most amazing race. I miss the partner I know and rely on. I miss the familiar routines and the times of being mobile with full knowledge that home base is being cared for. I have all these ideas about how to take care of Darryl. I am worried about the hospital bills. I am worried about our financial future. I am worried about my own health and the level of anxiety and stress I am feeling. Miracles can take a while, and I need the solid ground of optimism and of adventure. I really do not know what I am being asked to do right now. I just know that I can only take one day at a time. I try to be grateful for the beauty that surrounds me, and the love that we continue to have. The birds are singing in the dawn. The coffee is good.

Darryl spent nearly a month in the ICU; for much of the time, he had tubes in every natural orifice, as well as some manufactured ones. He left the ICU for a month-long stay in the rehabilitation unit, where he relearned how to talk, walk, and feed himself. Together we learned to get him bathed and dressed. After several long conferences with staff, we made plans for his return home.

Throughout Darryl's hospitalization, we received a tremendous amount of support from family, friends, and the hospital staff members, who were in a sense our family too. His friends at the fire department (where he had been a volunteer firefighter) held a fundraiser and remodeled our bathroom with grab bars and other assistive devices. A group of our coworkers gathered beside us as we left the hospital. They surrounded us with floating balloons and signs of good wishes. It was amazing. And then, I was on my own at the beginning of full-time caregiving.

Occupational therapists, speech therapists, and physical therapists came to our home for the first month or two. It seemed as if they were constantly in the house, asking about his progress, putting him through exercises, and giving me instructions for the exercises I needed to do with him. It was overwhelming. I went back to work in June, and our oldest son took leave from his work in order to be the daytime caregiver. By the end of June, we decided that Darryl could be left alone with frequent phone check-ins and a Life Alert bracelet. Each morning, I got him dressed, gave him breakfast, and set up a lunch for him before going to work. In the evening, I came home, fed the animals, cooked dinner, cleaned up the kitchen, and began the bedtime routine. Transportation to outpatient therapy was difficult due to lack of public transportation in the rural area where we live. It seemed that I was constantly juggling schedules and responsibilities for caregiving, homemaking, and work.

In those first months, I noted that Darryl often covered his feelings of inadequacy, or his mistakes, with laughter. The morning dressing process often was difficult, since it required getting his arms and legs in the right places. Once he started laughing at his difficulties, I could join in, and we both felt better. Then he started complaining about his clothes when they were hard to put on. He did not like sweat pants that had sheen; he called them "sleazy bastards." He has retained a few choice names for clothes that are difficult to get into or that he has some dislike for. He has always loved to tease and "fool" people, and I have often been his biggest fool. Sometimes, even now, it is hard to tell if he is teasing or if he is covering for a perceived deficit.

July 14, 2005

I want to run away. This is not my life anymore...at least I do not recognize its shape in some fundamental way. And yet, I do recognize it, like the shadow that has been waiting underneath the surface, the suffering that transforms the usual activities of daily life into a precious gift, a gift that is not pain-free, but still exquisite in its fleeting beauty.

I began to understand a little more about brain injury, not in any academic way, but in a very experiential way. Darryl asked me several times about his road bicycle; he was sure that it was in the barn. We looked repeatedly, and eventually decided it had been stolen out of the unlocked barn. I added locking the barn to my long list of chores. A few months later, I attended an awards ceremony for a coworker and gave him an update on Darryl's condition. He said, "If he has difficulty remembering who I am, tell him that I am the guy who bought his road bike." I stopped locking the barn.

October 10, 2005

I'm tired this morning, but grateful to be up early enough to sit and write for a bit. I sure do not get much done on the days I work, and I do not get much done on my days off because of appointments. I seem to bounce around one day feeling like a failure, the next day feeling joyful, and the next angrily trying to wrest control over an unruly inner and outer universe. I am reminded over and over about how easy it is to think that this present state of affairs will last indefinitely, of how surprised I am when things change, for better or for worse. I want to be filled with joy and confidence; more often than not, I am contracted and fearful.

Darryl had to have major surgery on his carotid artery at the end of 2005. He was in the ICU for a couple of days; during that time he was more alert and able to cooperate with the caregivers. What a way to end the frantic year.

In the early part of 2006, we flew to Mexico to stay with some dear friends in their time-share. We had a wonderful time visiting with them in Mexico, but it was not an easy trip. The logistics of travel, the crowds in the airport, and the unfamiliarity created a lot of anxiety for Darryl. He had to focus on walking while continuously asking where he was, and where he was going. I struggled with wanting the trip to be fun in the old familiar way and was disappointed about how much work it was for me. It was difficult to walk to nearby restaurants for dinner, and sightseeing was not at all comfortable.

Our friends took us on a boat tour to a lovely little village where we had lunch on the beach. There was no dock, so we were loaded into small motorboats for the trip to the beach. Darryl was able to get down into the motorboat, but with great difficulty. Loading him back into the boat from the surf was quite the scene. Our friend John and I literally picked him up and threw him into the boat. What a memory! Looking back, I realize how unrealistic my expectations were. We could not have done this trip without friends helping us and guiding us, but they were also a bit unrealistic about what Darryl could do for himself.

Friday, March 12, 2006

I think I expected Darryl to be more like his old self on this vacation. So yesterday, when he fell, he got real grumpy and told me that I was hovering too much. I was really disappointed. Actually, the disappointment has been happening for days.

I kept making decisions based on the man I used to know rather that the man he had become. This made both of us vulnerable to some unpleasant surprises. Darryl had always enjoyed helping others, so I decided that some volunteer work was in order. I signed us up to deliver Meals on Wheels. Soon he started refusing to deliver meals. He did not want to walk up to the door and visit with people. I felt it necessary to continue to deliver meals for several months without him. I also purchased an exercise bicycle based on what I thought would motivate him to return to his former self, but he never took to it. I can only see this in hindsight; at the time I believed that I was being helpful. It was frustrating for both of us.

Saturday, May 20, 2006

I realize that my expectations have to be altered of what Darryl may or may not be able to do. He may learn to do many more things than he can do right now, but my idea of his going back to doing things he once loved in the past is flawed. It seems I have many lessons to learn about being with him, where he is, and aligning with his strengths.

The difficulties of losing my partner to disease ran through my discussions with myself. I tried very hard to learn what I thought were the lessons I was supposed to learn, but I felt a sense of not being enough and not doing enough. I felt abandoned, tired, impatient—so many negatives. To make it worse, I tried to numb myself with alcohol or beat myself about the negatives. I have learned to try very hard not to compare my life to the lives of my friends. But sometimes I am still blindsided by what feels like intense envy.

After two years of unrelieved caregiving, I hoped that 2007 would be better, but it was not. I was still working, still feeling lonely but never alone, still trying hard to make things right for Darryl and for me. It was not working. I filled my thoughts of retiring from work in 2008 and hoped that life would become easier after retirement.

I was getting very tired and overwhelmed by the numerous daily chores, activities, and pressures of everyday life with a disabled person. First, I tried to figure out how to describe my loved one's condition. I usually said he was disabled, but it sounded so permanent. I wondered if I should say that he has an illness, is sick, or has a condition. Second, I didn't know how to phrase what I said in the presence of my loved one. The caregiving activities do not vary from day to day in terms of helping with dressing, bathing, cleaning glasses, fetching water, preparing and serving food, administering medications, monitoring ambulation, and answering questions and requests. Third, I was planning social events, which in our case involved asking friends or family to dinner or going out for some activities, which were both difficult for, and unwelcome by, Darryl. Additionally, all of the driving, all of the grocery shopping, all of the yard and farm work, and all of the housework became mine, as did decisions about house repairs and appliance break-downs. Unexpected events like falls, and assisting him to get up, kept me vigilant and on guard. Finally, late-night trips to the emergency room and unexpected illnesses and surgeries provoked an underlying but constant anxiety. It was like always waiting for the other shoe to drop.

I retired from paid work in June 2008. I had not expected such an adjustment to retirement. After a few months, I realized that I had traded caring for many patients, whom I felt that I was able to help, to caring for one patient, my husband, for whom I felt I had very little ability to help. I also had the mental habit of judging my accomplishments for the day based on the productivity expectations of my nursing career. It did not work. I felt like I was failing to take adequate care of my one patient.

Alcohol began to play a large part in my attempt to numb myself. I did not want to feel the anger, the help-lessness, the grief, and all of the other difficult emotions that go along with the life changes that I was experienc-ing. I felt robbed of the ability to have fun in retirement. I was unable to go places and do things that I had previ-ously enjoyed on my own. Alcohol numbed but did not change the feelings. Each evening I had a party by myself at home so that I could forget that I was not having any fun. I became frightened that I was doing damage to my body. As tired and miserable as I was, I did not want to abandon Darryl. Something had to change. I had a conversation with a dear friend who is in recovery. She guided me to Alcoholics Anonymous.

Sobriety brought many gifts into my life. At first, I noticed few changes. I was still angry, frustrated, frightened, and full of excuses and circular thinking. I started seeing a wonderful therapist, who began to help me unwind some of the tangled thinking that I had accumulated. She encouraged me to think about things differently and to take care of myself in ways that I had not been able to manage. The steps of Alcoholics Anonymous also guided me into healthier habits in my daily life.

Darryl continued to undergo physical changes, and most were not good. We often were in the doctor's office for miscellaneous complaints that were the result of major changes in his body and mind. He had the tip of one of his toes amputated because it folded under another toe, and it hurt when he walked. He had gall-bladder surgery. He had an appendectomy. He began to have more trouble walking and complained of knee pain. The pain was not relieved by cortisone injections or pain medications. Surgery was indicated, so he had a knee replacement. The recovery from that surgery was long, painful, and arduous. It seemed like we were locked in the house together for weeks, and it was winter, making our situation even more uncomfortable. And, of course, we had to spend time and energy going back to physical therapy appointments.

It took a long time, but it began to dawn on me that Darryl would not get well in the way that I had hoped. This realization was an insidious process that started without being put into words after the first year of our new life. I kept hoping that he would recover more function than he had. It was a lurch-forward, fall-back, trial-and-error kind of process. Somewhere toward the end of that first year of our journey, I began to understand that the area in Darryl's brain that managed initiation and motivation was permanently gone. I tried to make it OK by articulating that it kept him safe—that he could say he wanted to go out and drive the truck or tractor, but he could not initiate the activity. But his lack of motivation did not help with getting him to be independent in doing his exercises. I soon learned that it is difficult to be the motivator for someone else. Additionally, he began to have more poststroke symptoms in the affected side: more rigidity, more pain, and more stiffness. His ability to walk deteriorated slowly, as did his ability to dress himself. He could no longer make a peanut butter sandwich, or carry something from the microwave or refrigerator to his chair. His balance had also been affected by the brain injury, which made him at high risk for falling. Sometimes he would try to walk through things rather than around them. Obviously, his judgment had been affected.

One of the most difficult parts of being a full-time caregiver for a loved one is the inevitable irritation about petty things. Annoyances are just a part of life lived with another human being, but those involuntary and repetitive odd habits can really get to me. I always feel bad when I react with impatience; it is not like he is doing these things to irritate me. Another of the most difficult parts of this job as caregiver is the management of chronic pain. It seems like it is always something: knee pain, arm pain, ingrown toenail pain, back pain, and on it goes. I find my nurse self constantly feeling like a failure because I cannot make this one person who means so much to me even remotely comfortable.

In 2011 Darryl was diagnosed with esophageal cancer. This seemed like the final blow. He was not strong enough to tolerate both chemotherapy and radiation. He was very weak and unable to eat much. It appeared that he would be gone in a few months, given the severity of the disease. We opted for palliative radiation that would hopefully relieve the pain and make him more comfortable in his final months. Shortly after the cancer diagnosis, the Veteran's Administration awarded Darryl full disability for his heart disease. I had done the paperwork and shepherded his application for the disability months earlier, after learning that Agent Orange exposure in Vietnam was linked to ischemic heart disease. I felt somewhat comforted that neither Darryl nor I was responsible for the chain of disease that Darryl had sustained. The people who talked with Darryl at the VA thanked Darryl for the service that he had given for our country. I became patently aware that the war of our youth was still with us in tangible form. Inevitably, the wars we are presently fighting have dramatically and eternally changed the lives of people and their families who serve in the military today.

We were not sure what had happened with the cancer. Darryl has not had any symptoms since about six months after the initial diagnosis. He has regained all of the weight he lost and then some. We were grateful, and happily mystified.

In 2012, two days after my sixty eighth birthday, I had a heart attack, an unpleasant wake-up call. I was told in no uncertain terms by my family that it was time to hire some help with Darryl. I hired help two mornings a week and began to take a yoga class once a week. I also began to take small getaways for myself. Our children were able to spend the night with their dad when I took these little breaks. It was hard to ask the "kids" for their help, since they have very busy lives with their jobs and children. I tried to time my getaways with their busy schedules.

During this past year, I found a facility to take Darryl as a respite resident. I have enjoyed several weeklong breaks, and I have concluded that it is time for me to relinquish much of the responsibility I have carried for so long. Soon we will be moving from our home into an assisted-living facility. I am looking forward to having more time to pursue some neglected interests, to not cooking three meals a day, seven days a week, and not having the responsibilities for farm chores. I am so sad about leaving the home that I have been in for forty-four years, as well as the animals and the greenhouse. Our eldest son and his wife have bought the place, so it really is the best of both worlds. I can play in the dirt anytime I want without the chores of maintenance. It is a new beginning with new opportunities.

Although I initially described this as a love story, it is a far cry from being romantic. This love is hard working, patience testing, and sometimes gut wrenching. This love requires the willingness to be present to the joy and sorrow without becoming attached to either one, to simply let life flow and try to respond appropriately. This love requires a constant balancing between compliance and resistance, compassion and anger, and my needs and wants versus his needs and wants. Our friends and family have been willing helpers and open-hearted listeners. We could not have survived so well without their loving kindnesses and occasional kicks in the butt. I am grateful for all of them.

> *"In good times love is lovely. Nothing can be better. And in hard times, love is necessary. It turns tragedy into opportunity: something difficult and unwanted becomes a chance to drive love deeper, to make it wiser, fuller, more glorious, and more resilient."*
> *—Norman Fischer*

Two

Guilt: My Dysfunctional Family — Anonymous

Mother had been shouting and flailing her arms in the air when she pushed me out the door. As I ran past her, she screamed, "Go get your father right now! Tell him to get himself here, because I am going to be very sick! Go! Do you hear me?" I ran across the street to the tobacco warehouse where my father worked. Tears were streaming down my face as I ran into the building. I saw my dad, grabbed his hand, and pulled him toward the door. "Ma is sick, and she wants you to come home right now. Hurry, please."

He picked me up in his arms and ran across the street to the house. Mother was lying on the couch and moaning loudly. I stood by the door while Dad went to her side. I heard her say, "I tried to commit suicide. It is her fault. She made me do it." Feelings of guilt consumed my being.

I went out on the small, rambling porch and peeped through the screen door. I was shaking with fear as she revealed to Dad that she had swallowed something that was kept under the washstand in the kitchen. He knelt beside the couch, took both her hands, and told her that she was going to be OK. He told her not to cry. I stayed out on the porch until Dad came out almost an hour later. I started sobbing loudly and asked him if she was going to be all right. He assured me that she was going to be fine and that she needed to sleep now.

Dad left and went back to work. I remained on the porch until I heard Mother groaning and getting up to go to the outdoor privy. Within a few hours, she fully recovered from the ingredients that she had ingested. When I went into the house, there was vomitus all over the living room floor. She attempted suicide again within a year.

Lola and Eugene Jackson adopted me when I was one year old. The details of the adoption were never made clear to me. I learned that my biological mother gave birth to me when she was sixteen. She did not give the name of the biological father on the birth certificate. Lola was acquainted with both of my biological parents, who lived in or near the small town of Prairie du Chein (PDC), Wisconsin. I learned from a reliable source that my biological mother, Doris, had paid Lola one thousand dollars to take me. Little did Doris know that she was leaving her baby daughter with a very dysfunctional family, especially my Mother, Lola.

Lola and Eugene had no children of their own when they adopted me. When I was three, my brother Eugene was born. He was always Mother's favorite.

Mother told me that Dad had given her syphilis (STD) when they first married. When she became pregnant, she had the pregnancy interrupted because she was afraid the baby would be deformed. Throughout my childhood, I kept hearing her outbursts of anger toward him and her shouts of, "You gave me syphilis, you old fool! You have made my life miserable! I can never forgive you!"

Not long after the suicide attempt, I saw Mother standing by the wood stove, canning peaches. I walked up to her and pulled on her skirt to get her attention. "I want to see what you are doing, and I want a drink of water."

She stopped what she was doing and pushed me away from her.

"Can't you see that I am busy? You should not be around the hot stove and bothering me when I am working. I would like to throw you on the floor and smash your head in." Why did I always do or say the wrong thing? I was so frightened. I ran out of the house, got on my kiddy cart, and pedaled to Grandma Kent's house as fast as my thin, short legs would carry me.

Grandma Kent lived four blocks away. I had been told not to cross the two large streets in between, but I had to get away from my angry mother. I ran into the safety of the arms of my mother's mother. I loved my Grandma Kent very much. She was always there for me, and she soothingly dried my tears. She became my only retreat for several years.

These are some of the incidents that I recall from my early childhood. Many similar episodes followed, in which Mother showed her disdain and dislike toward me. Feelings of guilt became an overpowering force in my life. I still carry this tremendous sense of guilt that Mother instilled in me as a child and as a young adult. Why did she behave toward me in such a hostile manner? Of what am I guilty? It was always "that girl's fault" when something did not suit her or when she became frustrated with a particular situation. Was I such a dismal failure?

These incidents were fueled with Mother's anger, almost to the point of rage. From early childhood, I have had difficulty coping with individuals who express anger toward me. I learned to keep my feelings bottled inside. I could not share my feelings of frustration and inadequacies with either Mother or Dad, or with my few friends or other relatives—not even with my beloved Grandma Kent.

When Mother came home from the hospital with my little brother, the neighbors welcomed them both with presents. I recall standing at the foot of the bed in which my mother and her new son were resting. I hoped that the neighbors had brought me presents too, but they only patted me on the head and told me what a handsome brother I had. I ran out of the house, jumped on my kiddy cart, and pedaled over to Grandma Kent's house.

Mother kept Eugene in the bed in her bedroom and told Dad and me, "He likes to play with the hair under my arms." Mother continued to sleep with Eugene until he was teenager. I recall that I slept in a large crib in the same room with Mother and Eugene. Dad slept on a cot in a small adjoining room.

Mother would get up some nights and go into Dad's room. One night when I stood up in my crib and sang in a loud voice, "I know where you are going," she picked me up, took me out of the crib, and shook me violently. She began a verbal tirade with, "Now, you hush! And if you cry, I will smash you onto the floor!" I heard her tell Dad, "I just can't stand that girl." I was always "that girl." Later she told me that I had embarrassed her and that she stopped going to see Dad at night because I made her feel guilty.

I loved my Dad very much, and we did things together like fishing, hiking the beautiful hills around PDC, and going for excursions in the car on Sunday afternoons. He built me a cute little doll bed, a red chair, and a low seat for the outdoor privy.

Sometimes Mother treated me more like a sister than a child. One day she confided in me that she was pregnant. She also told me that I was not to tell any-one. I told my cousin James about what Mother had said and told him not to tell anyone. He told his mother, who immediately talked with Mother. She called me into the house and said, "You caused me to lose that baby because you told James. You were the cause of this. Why else would I lose the baby that I wanted so much? You were the cause. I would like to beat you." If she was pregnant, the actual father could have been one of several men about town. In addition, she may have contracted an STD from one of her many boyfriends.

I became a pimp at a very early age by carrying notes and messages to her numerous male friends. On one occasion, I recall that Mother had told me to get under the bed and take money from Mr. Masson's overall pockets when he got in bed with her. Mr. Masson came to the house almost every morning at a fairly early hour. I was under the bed when they started making lots of loud groaning and grunting noise and thrashing about during their sexual activity. I knew it was time to get as many coins as I could from the pockets when I heard Mother say, "Let's pretend that we are ponies running up and down the hills." The noises continued as I extracted the coins. I was sure that he could not hear me, so I quietly and quickly scooted across the bedroom floor and darted out of the room. It is unlikely that either of them knew that I had been present to hear the racing of the ponies. A few days later, I told some neighborhood kids about the under-the-bed experience. I did not know that Mother and her sister Faye were listening to my revelation of the racing ponies through a window just above where the group was gathered. Faye joined Mother in a lengthy session of verbal abuse while the other kids were still present. I was so humiliated. "That girl" always caused grief and pain.

After Faye and Mother were through with the raging verbal abuse, I became very angry and wanted to run away forever. I was cornered. I was trapped. I had no control over my life. My only outlet was to get on my bike and pedal as fast as my legs would go. I desperately needed to get away from this horrible, ongoing scene, but things just kept closing in on me. I felt so alone with all the anger that was continuously boiling up in me. I had no one with whom I could share these horrible feelings of being trapped.

I decided to ride my bike into town to get away from the stress and pressure that had become such an integral part of my everyday feelings. As I was pedaling down the street of downtown PDC, I noticed that one of the town's drunks was sitting in the street and throwing money at people as they passed by. I quickly dismounted from my bike and ran over to pick up several quarters, nickels, and dimes. I rushed back home to give the surprise to my mother.

When I gave the money to Mother, she became very angry because I had not picked up more money, particularly the paper money. She told me to get over to Mr. Matthew's house and ask him for some money. I felt that I had to do what she asked or face her agonizing verbal abuse and obvious anger. Mr. Matthew's blind sister finally answered the door after several knocks. I told her that my mother had sent me to speak to Mr. Matthew and that I needed to see him immediately. When Mr. Matthew came to the door, I told him who I was and that my mother wanted some money from him. He readily handed over a couple of one-dollar bills and told me to be sure to give them to my mother and to get out of there quickly. He was one of Mother's most frequent suitors. When I gave the money to Mother, she smiled and said, "You are such a good girl."

Mother and Dad argued almost constantly when he came home from work. The arguments were not about Mother's numerous boyfriends; instead they argued about money. She always wanted more money. The economic depression that was prevalent across the country had curtailed the number of jobs available. She did not realize how fortunate Dad was to have a job that at least allowed us to have the basic necessities.

During one of their heated arguments, a terrible verbal altercation ensued. Mother picked Eugene up and told Dad to get out and "take that girl with you." Dad left immediately without me, but he returned a week later. I never knew where he stayed when he left the house for several nights.

Soon thereafter Mother told me to take a note to Mr. Watson, who worked at the local hardware store. On the way to the store, I read the note. "You owe me money. I am raising your son without any help from you. I mean now." When I got back home, I looked at Eugene, my adoptive brother, and wondered if he really was Mr. Watson's son. I soon let go of that idea, as the shape of his face and his eyes resembled Dad's.

Another of Mother and Dad's heated arguments turned into a furious wrangle. Eugene and I were in the room listening to the angry exchange. Both of us were so scared that we could not move. I heard Dad call Mother a slut. She walked right up to his face but stopped when their noses almost touched. She put her hands on her hips and started screaming at Dad. In a loud screeching voice, Mother yelled at him, "You are an idiot, a weakling, and a moneyless good-for-nothing! I never want to see you again! And take that girl with you! I want you both out of this house!" She ran over to Eugene and picked him up and continued shouting, "Out, out, both of you out!" Dad turned toward me and smiled. He left the house without me. I had never felt so alone, and I wanted to run to him. I was so glad to see him when he eventually returned. I felt that he really cared for me, and he kissed me good-night in my bed.

Several times Mother left Dad for other men. One such sexual escapade was with a man called "little carpenter." He was probably given that name because of his small stature and his trade. The man's daughter sent a letter to Mother, and she shared the letter with me. The letter said, "If you don't leave my father alone, I will get a lawyer to take legal action against you."

I do not think Mother ever saw the little carpenter again, at least not during the daytime. She often left the house at night for a couple of hours. I would sit up to wait for her. When she came home, she would do a quick hand-douche with Lysol and water. She never bothered to give Dad or me an explanation for her absence. Even as a kid, I knew that she was screwing around with a lot of men. She manipulated me into being a go-between for her and her sexual suitors.

One of Mother's most frequent and attentive male visitors was Mr. Donahue. I saw him walking past the house almost daily. I also noticed that Mother would put notes under a can when she knew that he would be walking by. One day I slipped out of the house and read the note that she had placed under the can. The note was asking for money.

Although most of her sexual escapades were about money and with married men, a few of them seemed to be about manipulating men and enticing them into her larkish games. She bragged to me about trying to seduce my cousin James (her nephew) when he was a teenager. She laughingly told me that he was not able to "put out." Likewise, she tried to seduce Jason, my biological mother's nephew, who owned a grocery store in town. She told me that she just couldn't help herself when she was "around all of this good beef."

Grandma Kent soon became a haven of security for me. Her mother, who was one hundred years old, visited her often. She was a small, stooped woman, and I liked her very much. I identified with her because she seemed to be so lonely. When anyone would ask me how old I was, I would think of my great grandmother and add my actual age to one hundred. She suddenly stopped coming to visit her daughter, and I learned that she had become disabled and died shortly thereafter. I am thankful for the short time that we had together.

I stayed with Grandma Kent for a year when Dad's tobacco company sent him to Pennsylvania. Mother and Eugene went with him. At first I felt abandoned when the three of them left me. During my year with Grandma Kent, however, I found a new lease on life. I realized that I was growing up in a nice, caring environment in which there were no verbal hassles or angry outbursts from Mother.

When the year was over, the four of us, Mother, Dad, Eugene, and I, moved back into our old house in PDC, but we had much less room. Mother had rented out one-half of the house to a couple in order to get additional money during the depression. She also started selling Avon products, and when they arrived through the mail, I would deliver the items to customers on my bike. I decided that I could be an Avon sales clerk, and I started selling and delivering the products on my own. Of course, Mother took most of the money that I made.

She soon reverted back to her numerous men friends for money.

The family situation became even more intense when Grandma Kent died. We moved in with Grandpa Kent so that Mother could take care of him. Money had become even sparser as the economic depression continued. Dad's job as a sales clerk at the tobacco company required that he be out of town during the week, so he was only home on weekends. I looked forward to his weekend visits, but I knew that Mother only tolerated his presence. She could put up with almost anything as long as the money kept coming in.

Along with her indiscreet sexual activities, Mother tried to turn me against Dad. One summer night, we were out on a hill gazing at the stars. Mother said she was going to make a wish. She began the refrain, "Star light, and star bright. First star I see tonight. I wish I may, I wish I might, have the wish I wish tonight." She then told me that she wished Dad would die, and she asked me to make the same wish. I was so scared, but I kept my thoughts to myself. I wished that the next day would be a nice day.

Grandpa Kent became ill while we were living with him. He complained of constant nausea and acute abdominal pain. He refused to eat the food that Mother fixed for him, and then he started to feel better. Mother told me that she had been putting small pieces of castor bean in his food. I later learned that castor beans were poisonous. Mother said that she did this because Grandpa Kent was sexually active with a neighbor woman.

One day, while living with Grandpa Kent, Mother gave me some letters to mail along with money for stamps. I got on my bike and went to the post office in town. Much to my dismay, I discovered that I had lost the money that Mother had given me for stamps. What could I do? I quickly pedaled back to Grandpa's house and told him of my plight. I asked him if he would give me the money to pay for the stamps. He said, "Yes, if you will get into my lap."

I was bewildered and did not want to sit in his lap, but I had to get some money for the stamps or face Mother's furious rage. So I got into his lap. Soon he was unbuttoning my blouse and putting his old withered, whiskered face on my breasts. I tolerated it for a few minutes and then jumped down. He said, "I'm just a lonesome old man. I won't hurt you."

I was crying as I ran out of the house. I grabbed my bike and went back to the post office. It took me years to get over the feeling of his old whiskered face on my breasts. Feelings of guilt over what happened washed over me. I never told anyone of this incident. Thank goodness we moved out of his house soon thereafter.

Even now, as I recall that incident with Grandpa, I wonder if he molested Mother and her two sisters, Faye and Lillie, when they lived at home with him (their father). I sometimes speculate that Mother was using sex with numerous married men as a vehicle to get back at her father for what he possibly did to her. Mother was a very attractive woman, and she could probably have had her pick of men. But for some unknown reason, she chose to flaunt herself and allow men to use her at their will. She was almost six feet tall and a little on the heavy side. She had beautiful dark hair and developed a taste for attractive clothes. While this is only speculative thinking after many years, my episode with Grandpa has often made me wonder if her father's behavior with her might have influenced Mother's choices in life.

We moved into a small apartment near the railroad tracks when we left Grandpa's house. The bed bugs were so bad that I either slept on the balcony off the bedroom or in Dad's car that was parked near the railroad tracks. The tramps that lived in the same area never bothered me.

We eventually moved back to our old home across from the tobacco warehouse. Space was at a premium, though, because the couple that had moved in retained one-half of the house. The tensions that had become such an integral part of our family relationships only intensified.

Even with all of the hateful and mean things that Mother said and did to me, I was always afraid of losing her. I tried to do everything to please her, and I abstained from anything that I thought would incur her wrath.

Despite all my efforts, however, I always inadvertently seemed to become a victim of her anger and abuse.

Out of this disparaging sea of hopelessness, a propitious event occurred that altered my remaining life. When I was in the fourth grade, I was getting a drink at the water fountain at school when a classmate shoved my head into the water spigot. The bottom part of my two front teeth was knocked off. I went to the teacher, and she asked about my parents. During the conversation, she asked if I was adopted. After I replied, "Yes," she told me that she thought she knew who my biological father was. "I think your father is Roy Fancher. You are the spitting image of Roy. I know his parents, and they live over in Bloomington."

After some discussion with Mother, the Fanchers were notified of my whereabouts. They were overwhelmingly surprised that I was still alive. My biological mother had sent them a letter almost ten years previously saying that I had died and asking for money for my burial. They readily complied with her request for money. Upon learning that indeed I was alive and well, they insisted on seeing me. Mother readily arranged for the meeting.

I could not believe that I was the granddaughter of this attractive older man and woman and a niece of the two exceedingly attractive young women who were my aunts. They each welcomed me warmly and told me that Roy, my biological father, had married and lived in Cassville, which was a small town about thirty-five miles away. Each of the aunts said that they wanted to keep in touch with me and would welcome some time to get to know me better. They would be in touch with Roy and knew that he would want to see me. They would make all the arrangements after contacting him. What a joyous moment in my troubled life!

Arrangements were made for me to visit Roy and his wife. They seemed glad to see me but did not leave me with the profuse feelings of belonging that I had with his parents and sister. While I was visiting, I overheard Roy say to his wife that he had not married Doris (my biological mother) because he did not love her. He then said his name was not on the birth certificate but that he could take me from my adoptive parents whenever he wanted to.

I was absolutely devastated when I heard Roy say that he had not married my biological mother because he did not love her. I had always told my friends that I was a love child. I still wonder what their mothers said to them when they asked, "What is a love child?"

When I got back home, Mother assured me that she would never allow Roy to take me away from her. I believed her, even though she never really seemed to care for me. She expected me to be home right after school to do the numerous chores around the house. While I was emptying the ashes from the wood-burning stove and chopping more wood for the always-needy woodpile, my brother was glued to the radio, listening to all the kids' shows that came on in the evening. Mother's behavior toward me was obviously less positive and more punitive than her behavior to my brother. However, I was still afraid of losing her.

When I was still in junior high school, Mother, Eugene, and I moved to Beloit, Wisconsin, to live with her new man friend and his family of seven children, five of whom still lived at home. There were nine of us packed in a house with one bedroom, a living room, a bathroom, and a kitchen. Of course, Mother and Mr. Gardner got the bedroom. During the summer, most of us slept outside on the porch or on the ground. I never had a moment of privacy with all the people coming and going day and night.

After about a year, Eugene and I insisted that we move away from the Gardner family. We moved a few blocks away into a small, one-room house that was nearer to the high school. I strung up a sheet in a corner of the room, put a mattress on the floor, and put my few belongings, including my clothes, in a cardboard box from the grocery store. Mr. Gardner was still around, but at least I had my own space. I rarely saw my Dad, but he always came around at Christmas and gave me nice presents of jewelry, scarves, and books.

I was not at all popular in high school and had very few friends and few dates. I did not feel attractive and rarely smiled. Grandma Kent had told me several years ago that I would be quite attractive if I would smile. I do not know if it was because I had a space between my two front teeth (inherited from the maternal side of my family) or because I was so unhappy. It was probably both.

World War II was in full swing while I was a senior in high school. The days of school each week were reduced to four. Like most of my fellow students, I took a job as a clerk at the local Woolworth's five and dime store. From my meager earnings, I bought all of my clothes and gave some money to Mother each week.

I graduated from Beloit High School in the upper 5 percent of the class. I continued my job at the local Woolworth's. We moved into a larger house, and Mother took in four male boarders. Most of the responsibility of cleaning, cooking, and keeping the house in order was left to me. I had little time to get together with my two or three girlfriends or to date the few boys who were hesitant to come to the house.

Mother told me that she had always wanted to become a nurse and that one of her fondest dreams was for me to become a nurse. I had been out of high school for one year when I received a scholarship for the entry fee to a nursing school of my choice from a women's association in Beloit. I applied to several schools and willingly accepted the offer from Milwaukee General Hospital.

At last I was able to escape from the entrapment that I had been in for most of my life. I never regretted the move away from Mother and her almost constant wrathful behavior toward me. I vowed that I would never live with her again. Mother told me some years later, "It broke my heart when you left me." I still find that hard to believe. She no longer had me to blame for her flagrant behavior.

When I left Beloit, Eugene moved back to PDC to finish high school. He lived with a family that had been friends of Dad's for many years. Dad still lived in PDC and became a stable force in Eugene's life. Like me, Eugene had suffered the traumatizing aftermath of existing in an extremely dysfunctional family.

I felt as if I had been reborn when I moved to Milwaukee to enter the three-year nursing education program. The changes were so welcome! At last, I became an awakened, vibrant individual. The past was behind me, and the future seemed to be a beckoning light that drew me out of my unsmiling face and introverted behavior. I made friends easily and soon became quite popular with other students; I was even elected president of the senior class. I was exceedingly excited when lots of guys started calling me for dates. I became engaged to Duncan and took him to meet Mother. She told me that it was OK with her if I never got married.

I soon broke my engagement with Duncan because I perceived him to be controlling like my mother, and he was becoming increasingly dependent on me (like my mother), and because he wanted to have children. I had vowed in my early teens that I would never have children. I had told Mother that I thought that I was pregnant because two of my adoptive cousins had slipped into my bedroom one night and tried to have sex with me. Mother told me that she would help me care for the baby. The act was not consummated, but I did not know then what was necessary to become pregnant. I learned this later in nursing training.

Duncan, the boy to whom I was engaged, wanted a large family, and he thought it was selfish of me to deny him that privilege. He made me feel like he wanted me only to have his babies.

There was another issue related to why I did not want a baby. Mother often talked with me about my biological mother, but never in glowing terms. On one occasion, she told me that Doris, my birth mother, had been going with a black shoeshine man in PDC when she was pregnant, and that I was probably the child of this man. I broke into tears and proclaimed, "I will never have a baby because I might have black genes." Mother did not respond to my outburst.

While in nursing training, I learned that Doris could not be pregnant with another fetus if she were already pregnant. Thus, I was able to discount another fallacy that Mother had maliciously implanted in my mind. Additionally, pictures of Doris indicated that she was attractive with very blond hair. Like my biological father, I had very dark hair and dark skin.

World War II had ended by the time I finished the three-year nursing program. My previous commitment to the cadet nursing corps, a wartime program that I had joined, and for which I had received thirty-five dollars per month for three years, was no longer obligatory. I readily took a position as a clinical nursing arts instructor at Milwaukee General Hospital. I moved out of the dorm and into an apartment.

Dad had moved back to Beloit after retirement. He became ill and was diagnosed with lung cancer. Mother moved back in with him and took care of him while she worked in a shoe factory. I went to see Dad when he was admitted to the hospital. I was able to tell him that I loved him and thanked him for everything he had done for me. He smiled and said, "It was never enough." My visit with Mother before and after his funeral was strained and uncomfortable.

I moved to Minneapolis, where I enrolled in the School of Public Health at the University of Minnesota. I earned a BS degree in public health nursing and an MPHN/mental health while working in the community health field as a teaching instructor.

True to their word, both of my biological aunts kept in touch with me through nursing training and college. Both of them had married, and Aunt Viola sent me pictures of her and her husband and their three children. We started corresponding more regularly when the family moved to Indianapolis, where her husband worked. I became very fond of both Aunt Viola and Aunt Dottie, and we had some great times together through the years. I felt their caring, love, and concern, and I appreciated their willingness to include me as a member of the Fancher family. They truly became "family" to me.

I wrote to my biological mother's sister to let her know of my academic accomplishments. I had hoped that the sister would share my letters with Doris so that perhaps she could be proud of her daughter. After sharing with the sister that I had received a master's degree from the University of Minnesota, she wrote back that Doris had married, had children, and did not want me to contact her again. I complied with her request. Much later, one of Doris's nieces shared pictures of the family with me. I saw a striking resemblance to my maternal grandmother.

While living in the St. Paul/Minneapolis area, Mother called and wanted to come and live with me. Without any hesitation or excuses, I told her absolutely not. Again, she was again furious with me and said I had no appreciation for all that she had done for me. I, however, felt that I had no obligation toward her and that I had done my duty for her.

She told me that she was living in Beloit and was supporting my brother, Eugene, who was married and had three daughters. She needed to get out of the situation. Soon thereafter she responded to ads in a magazine in which several men were advertising for a wife. The first man that came to see her was a schoolteacher, and he soon told her that he could not marry her because of her living situation with her son and his family. She married the second responder after receiving a one-thousand-dollar dowry from him. She was able to pay off Eugene's numerous debts that he had accumulated.

Mother's new husband, Arthur, was quite obese; he weighed over three hundred pounds. He had a big abdominal flap that hung down almost to his knees. He was hardly able to move around. Mother had to assist him with all of his activities of daily living. When I visited them, she seemed to be content and was affectionate toward him. She told me that he could not have sex because of the huge abdominal flap. She told me also that she no longer had sexual encounters with other men.

Mother moved back in with Eugene and his family after Arthur died. Even after I moved to Arizona, I drove back to Beloit during the summer to spend a week or two with her. We spent most of our time reminiscing about the past. I told her of a recurring dream that I had when I was seven or eight years old. In my dream, I was always alone in a park with lots of shrubs and bushes. I was holding a large stick and walking around whacking the bushes. Suddenly, I noticed an odor of sexual activity. I retreated when people started coming out of the bushes. I usually woke up at this point.

I told Mother that I had the dream again when I was a teenager. The dream occurred after I was changing the bedding from a cot in which one of our female boarders and her boyfriend had slept. As I was changing the linens, I smelled this strong odor of sex. The bushwhacking dream never occurred after that.

While visiting with Mother through the years, I realized that I had emulated her behavior in several ways. She had the habit of biting her nails, and I did the same until I went away from home. In addition, like Mother, I had sexual affairs with married men. The first was a one-night stand with a fellow that I met at a party. We had both been drinking. Somehow, somewhere, we ended up having sex—my first male encounter. I cried for days afterward. The second was with a psychiatrist who had erectile dysfunction, and the third was with a physician who told me that he had had a vasectomy. There were no babies.

I have had to work myself out of being entrapped after being adopted into a very dysfunctional family, primarily my adoptive mother. She was verbally abusive toward me. She was usually hostile toward me, and she was rarely kind or comforting to me. She used me as her pimp for most of my childhood. She used me as a chore girl during my teens. I have never been able to understand why she adopted me in the first place, except for the one thousand dollars from my biological mother.

I coped with feelings of being trapped by keeping my thoughts to myself; I did not share with anyone the feelings that I harbored toward Mother. I was a loner. I despised myself because I felt Mother despised me. I rarely smiled—I had nothing to smile about. I disengaged from family, friends, and neighbors that could have helped me if I had let them know what was happening. I was too ashamed and embarrassed to share what I was feeling. I had the bewildering bushwhacking dreams until my midteens.

Then I was offered the opportunity and had the good judgment to leave home and become a nurse. My academic and professional achievements have alleviated the barriers that kept me cornered for many years. In addition, most of all, I was able to respond with a profound "no" when Mother wanted to come and live with me. I did not want to feel the guilt that had cornered me during my formative years. Never again, ever.

Three

Living in the Present: A Stroke Survivor – Rosemary Johnson

On the evening of October 3, I was walking around the front yard of my house with Rosie, my dog, and feeling the gentle breeze that often comes with the beginning of autumn. I looked up at the beautiful log house that Judy, my friend of many years, and I had invested in more than eighteen years ago. We both had fallen in love with the house, the large one-acre yard, and the quiet, spacious neighborhood. I had planned and coordinated the landscaping of the entire acreage, and I felt appreciated when neighbors commented that the yard was beautifully composed. As I looked to the west, where the sun was beginning to set, I could see the towering peaks of the colorful red stones of the Granite Mountains that captured the sun's rays. What a glorious scene!

Judy called to me to come out on the backyard deck, where we retreated for our traditional evening cocktail. It was not unusual to hear a cacophony of crickets in the evening, or mating calls from the mourning doves earlier in the day. More than one hundred trees grew in our yard, attracting an abundance of deer, rabbits, quail, javelina, and coyotes. Occasionally a bushy-tailed fox would run through the yard. While we sat rocking back and forth in the porch swing, the stars started illuminating the sky. The enveloping darkness enhanced the brilliance of the stars. Honey, the cat, and Rosie, the dog, joined us for this quiet time together. I felt fine, loving, and full of life.

The next morning I heard an alarm going on and on, but I could not find the clock. After what seemed like hours, I heard Judy calling, "Maria, Maria, it's half past seven." I thought it was late evening and I was just awakening from a nap.

Judy came into the bedroom and turned the radio alarm off. She kept talking to me, but it seemed like she was some distance away. I could not understand what she was saying. I felt her touching my right arm and leg. I then heard her say, "Maria, hold out your left arm." I tried to understand what she wanted me to do. I heard her say again, "Maria, hold out your left arm." She then asked me to straighten out my left leg. I heard the words, but I did not know how to respond. Then I heard her say, "Maria, I think you have had a stroke. I am going to call

911." Her voice sounded miles away as I heard her speaking into the phone.

I felt her hands as she reached under my back. I could feel her moving my right arm from under my body. The bedside lamp was shining in my eyes, so I closed them. I felt Rosie jump up on the bed and nuzzle my arm to pet her, but I could not seem to move it. I felt another movement next to my head. Honey plopped herself down on my pillow. Everything was so very strange. I wanted to pet them both, but I could not make the movements. I closed my eyes and tried to figure out what time it was and where I was. In the far distance, I heard Judy say that emergency assistance was on its way. I could not think clearly; I tried to talk, but no words came out of my mouth.

I felt someone moving my arms and legs and rolling me over on my back. Whoever it was kept asking me to do things, but I could not understand what they were saying. I tried to keep my eyes open, but they kept closing to shut out the bright light in the room. I felt someone prop me up in bed, but I could only hear indistinct noises as they moved my body around.

Then I felt them put me on a stretcher and strap me down. I have no idea how much time elapsed before I heard the shrill wailing of a siren. I heard a muffled voice say, "We are taking you to the emergency room at the hospital." I was aware of being in an ambulance, and I tried to think through the route they were taking to the emergency room. *Let's see now...we are turning onto Treetops*

Drive, and after a couple more turns, we will be on Jacksonville Road. The siren was screaming as we sped down Rivers Road and up to the emergency room entrance.

The next thing I recall was lying on a gurney in the emergency room. I heard several voices, but I could not ascertain what they were saying. After an indefinite lapse of time, I recognized Judy's voice and felt her holding my hand. I opened my eyes but could not understand what she was saying. There seemed to be a lot of noise and movement around me. I had no comprehension of where I was or who was talking to me. I learned later that I had spent six hours lying on my back in the emergency room before being moved to a hospital room. I was told that I had spent seventy-two hours in the acute hospital. Nurses, doctors, and therapists were in and out of my room almost constantly. It was all a blur to me. Judy told me of her numerous visits, but I do not remember any of them.

I became aware that I was in a strange bed and that the room seemed to be dark. Where was I? How had I gotten there, and when had I arrived? Someone, perhaps it was Judy, told me that I was in a rehab hospital and that I was going to be there for three weeks while different therapies were administered. Various individuals told me at several different times that I had had a massive cerebral vascular accident a few days ago. I heard strange noises coming from my mouth. I did not know what I was saying, but I could hear myself trying to talk. It was as if I were in a dense fog and there was only a dim light for me to view my strange new environment. I did not remember having a stroke or the few days that I spent in the acute hospital following the stroke. Everything was so confusing. What was happening to me?

Therapy began abruptly on Monday morning. An occupational therapist came in at 7:00 a.m. and laboriously assisted me into the nearby bathroom. She had to physically extract me from the wheelchair, place me on the commode, and lift me back into the wheelchair. My left arm was flaccid and immovable, and I had no feeling in my left leg. Under her direction, and with her assistance, I was able to complete a sponge bath using my right hand. She then assisted me with dressing. "Always start with pulling the sleeve of your blouse over your bad arm. Pull it all the way up to your shoulder with your right hand. Now pull it over your head, and then put your right arm in the sleeve. Pull the blouse down now." She gave me short directions, one at a time. The first time the process of putting on my knit blouse took over fifteen minutes. It took another fifteen minutes for her to pull my sweat pants up and over the Depends underpants. Finally, she put on my socks and shoes. At 8:00 a.m., she pushed me in the wheelchair to the dining room and parked me at an assigned table. An aide brought me a glass of some kind of liquid and put a bib over my chest. I took small sips of the awful-tasting liquid. A nurse came in with my morning medications. It took me about ten minutes to take the pills because I had difficulty swallowing. This same process was repeated five days a week for the next three weeks. I was gradually able to follow directions more easily, and I started participating more in my toileting, bathing, and dressing. It was all such an effort, and my early recollections are quite vague.

Promptly at 9:00 a.m., a physical therapist came to take me to the activity center. The first day she did a series of evaluations. She explained that physical therapists would be working on my balance, muscle strengthening, coordination, and range of motion on my left side. The goal was to assist me in walking. I would start the ambulating process by standing, and then I was to proceed to walking between parallel bars. The therapist had to extract me from the wheelchair and lift me to a standing position. I was not able to balance myself, and I feared that I would fall. The therapist assured me that she was holding onto me, and after a couple of minutes, she lowered me back into the wheelchair. How would I ever walk between the parallel bars?

The first week I was placed on a treatment table, and a therapist conducted range-of-motion and passive muscle-strengthening exercises, particularly on my left side. I was given frequent instructions to pay more attention to what I was doing and try not to be distracted. I tried so hard to focus, but my concentration was shot.

During the middle of the second week, I was able to take a few faltering steps between the parallel bars. With each step, the therapist would instruct me to pick up my left foot and move it forward. My left hand kept slipping off the bars, and I would almost fall to the left before the therapist caught me. She would put my hand back on the bars and then asked me to stand up straight and continue with a few more steps. Feelings of utter dependence often overwhelmed me.

By the end of the third week, I was able to walk to the end of the bars and back, but only with constant supervision and assistance. The physical therapists had patiently assisted me in ambulating for very short distances and had helped me to restore some of my awkward balance. After each of the hourly sessions, they would take me back to the room and assist me in getting into bed. I was utterly exhausted after each session.

Speech therapy sessions started at 11:00 a.m. and went through the lunch period until 1:00 p.m. After an initial evaluation, Emmy, the speech therapist, told me we would be working on my facial drooping and speech problems during the first hour, and we would be going into a special dining room to work on my swallowing problems during the second hour. Each of these sessions was very intense. Emmy kept reminding me to swallow slowly when we were in the dining room, or to stay focused while working on puzzles that she gave me to test my cognitive abilities. It was so hard to concentrate, and I had no clear understanding of what I was being asked to do most of the time.

I soon realized how dependent I was becoming, not necessarily by choice, but by orders. I became so frustrated when people kept saying to me, "Don't be so distracted." I tried to follow all the orders, and I wondered why the therapists did not comprehend my efforts.

Emmy was very patient with me and engaged me in daily conversations about my career, my friends, my living arrangements, and my feelings about what was happening to me. Along with assisting me with my dysphasia and swallowing problems, she helped me to minimally understand the tremendous damaging effects of the stroke. She explained to me that I had to concentrate, to focus my brain on a leg, an arm, or any other body part I was trying to use. Why had no one told me that in the beginning rather than always ordering me not to be distracted? The fifteen sessions with Emmy not only helped me with problems associated with the stroke, but she also helped me learn to cope with my almost dysfunctional body and mind. It seemed to me that a lot of rehab time had been misused by giving me orders to not be distracted. Instead, they should have simply asked me to concentrate on the mind-body connection.

I hated the semiprivate room in which I had been placed. My revolving roommates and their visitors were usually quite noisy. I had the nurse pull the curtain between the beds, but that only made the dreary room even darker. There was one overhead television at the foot of the two beds, but I could not remember how to turn the TV on and off. My roommate sometimes asked what program I would like to see, but I had to defer to her choices since I did not know the program options. My biggest limitation and my overwhelming frustration was the complete loss of the use of my left hand. There was no feeling in that hand. One day I had a fantasy that if I could chop off my left hand, I would progress faster. I soon gave up that fantasy, since I knew how unrealistic it was.

Yet they expected me to learn to walk with a cane and to dress and undress myself. I was encouraged to swallow the food that they brought to me even though it had been ground into mush. I choked on foods that had not been pulverized. My speech was impaired, but I could carry on a little conversation. My thought processes were a bit garbled at times. I had difficulty using the cell phone that Judy left for me. I had always been very physically active and agile. Now I was wearing a diaper for incontinence and a bib to protect my clothes when I ate. I had been reduced to an infantile state. I was downright miserable and had difficulty understanding what had happened to me and why I was in this strange place.

Thoughts that kept chasing through my mind had to do with my extreme loss of independence. I had to become more dependent on others during the process of trying to restore my independence. I could not understand where this circular thinking was leading me. I would awaken at night trying to figure out how my dependence on others could increase my independence. I always came up with the same answer. Something had happened to me. I was no longer independent, as I had been most of my eighty-seven years. Now I could no longer drive my car or prepare a meal for myself. I could not even dress myself or walk the short distance to a bathroom. I had little feeling in my left arm and leg, and neither of them seemed to respond when I wanted them to. Whether independent or dependent, I was so very miserable and wanted my previous tranquil life back. Why did this happen to me?

There were some bright spots during my stay at the rehab hospital. Several friends dropped by for short visits, and they were so welcome. Particularly important were two Sundays when my friends Katrina, Grace, and Judy brought Rosie to see me for an hour. Judy wheeled me out to a picnic table behind the hospital, and Rosie was up in my lap before I was through the door. She was heavy and rambunctious, but I loved it. They had brought treats for me to feed her. We spent the hour watching her run around the enclosed area. I was unable to express adequately my profuse feelings of thanks for my friends' kindnesses.

I recall being wheeled into a conference room one morning during my third week at the facility. Several of the therapists, a social worker, and Judy were there. They told me that they had done all that they could for me. I needed to select a skilled nursing facility for the next phase of my rehabilitation. I should plan to move out in a few days.

I gave my thanks and good-byes to all the therapists and nurses that had led me through the tumultuous journey of return to reality. An ambulance moved me to a skilled nursing facility that Judy and the social worker had selected. Joy, joy, I had a private room with sunlight pouring in through the windows!

Therapy started at 6:00 a.m. with an occupational therapist assisting me with bathing and dressing. She then wheeled me to the dining room for breakfast, and I sat at an assigned table with two other patients. Physical therapy, which consisted of assisted ambulation between parallel bars and transferring from chair to commode and back, was conducted in an exercise room for over an hour. The physical therapist also gave me instructions on guiding the wheelchair. I usually had a nap after lunch and then dinner at 6:00 p.m. An occasional speech therapist dropped by for a short visit and left crossword puzzles for me to complete. I rarely completed any of the puzzles. I enjoyed Judy's visits and those from other friends.

I settled into a scheduled routine fairly well. I fell a couple of times when I tried to go to the bathroom unassisted. I so wanted to be independent. The lectures that followed were worse than the pain from the falls. Everyone kept telling me to pay attention to what I was doing. The nurses told me that I was never, never to get out of bed or out of the wheelchair without assistance. Judy, too, was concerned and gave me the same instructions. Oh, how I hated those constant demands. "Watch what you are doing. Do not get so distracted. Get assistance before getting out of the wheelchair or bed." I felt trapped by my own body and mind. I had lost all control over my being.

It was a relief when a team conference was held to evaluate my progress during the previous six weeks at the skilled nursing facility. I heard them say that I could plan to return home at the end of January. The occupational therapist arranged a home visit with Judy. Alterations would be made in the house so that when I came home, I could move about with a cane and wheelchair. In six weeks, I would be going home!

After being at the facility for a short time, I realized that I was tensing up. During one of the visits with Katrina, I confessed that I was feeling guilty about my stroke. I told her that I had left Judy with a tremendous responsibility as my healthcare power of attorney and as my durable power of attorney. Fiduciary and property care responsibilities were particularly burdensome. Katrina's response was that I should not feel guilty because I did not cause myself to have the stroke. Despite her reassurance, I could not erase the overpowering feelings of guilt that I had robbed Judy of several months of her life and that I was becoming a burden for her.

The holidays gave me additional time with my caring friends. I invited Judy to join me for Thanksgiving dinner at the facility. A few days later, a group of friends addressed holiday cards for me. Betty and Angie were my guests for Christmas dinner. The prospect of going home soon was the best gift that I could ask for.

On December 30, I gathered with several friends in the facility's activity room to celebrate my eighty-seventh birthday. Someone brought a beautiful cake with candles. Others had brought ice cream and snacks. The room was decorated with colorful tablecloths, and balloons floated in the air. Such wonderful friends made my day so memorable! I could not thank them enough for all their love, kindnesses, and attention.

Two days later, I tried to go to the bathroom by myself, and my left leg gave way. I took a hard fall and was unable to get up from the floor. A visitor from across the hall heard me calling and got an aide to lift me back into bed. The head nurse came in, checked me over for cuts and bruises, and told me that my blood pressure was high. She explained that it was facility policy for her to notify my guardian. Judy called later to see if I was all right. I had difficulty finding the right words to explain what had happened and that I was having some pain in my left hip. I asked her not to visit and told her that I would see her the next day. That was my celebration for the New Year of 2012. A nurse practitioner from Dr. Gates's office examined me the next day and ordered medication for pain.

The following morning was a nightmare. When I awakened, I did not know where I was. I called for Rosie, repeatedly, but she never came. Therefore, I called Judy but she never came. Eventually, an aide heard me and went for help. The head nurse called Dr. Gates. He discontinued the medication that the nurse practitioner had ordered for pain. My experience had been a horrendously frightening nightmare. I became so afraid of any medications after this incident.

It took several days for me to recover from the fall and from the hallucinations that followed the ingestion of the medication. I had been assigned to bed rest indefinitely. A nurse practitioner from Dr. Gates's office visited a few days later and ordered blood work, some new medications for my hypertension, and a reduction in therapeutic activities for the next few days. I began to wonder if I would be going home in three weeks as planned. I had not suffered any obvious physical damage from the fall, but I had been scared beyond words.

After more than a week, I was back to the previous regime of occupational therapy and physical therapy. It was obvious that I had lost ground during that span of time, but the passive exercises that they had conducted with me during the past week saved me from losing more of my earlier progress. It was back to bathing and dressing at 6:00 a.m., breakfast in the dining room at 7:00 a.m., and physical therapy later in the morning or early afternoon. I was using a walker to ambulate while the therapist held onto a gait belt to keep me from falling. I had learned to maneuver the wheelchair with some difficulty. It always veered to the left because I could use only my right hand. It took me at least thirty minutes to go from my room to the dining room for dinner. Fortunately, staff assisted me to breakfast and lunch and back to my room after dinner.

Friends continued to visit me, and on Sundays, Grace and Katrina brought my dog, Rosie, in to see me. My bond with my dog was weakening. When she initially saw me, during the visit, she was very excited, but her excitement did not last long. She went to Grace after a few minutes so that she could explore the room. Still it was good to see her and know that she remembered me.

Judy told me about all of the changes that had been made in the house so I could do more things for myself. She also had been exploring and arranging for special services from agencies that would provide home health care when I came home.

The day finally arrived for me to be discharged, and I would be able to go back home! My farewell to the able staff was both sad and happy. They each had been more than supportive in their continuous efforts to reach our goal of increased independence. It was good to sit in Judy's car as we drove over familiar territory to our home. The welcome that my friends gave me was only exceeded by the exuberance that Rosie displayed when I first entered the house. I slowly looked at the lovely log walls of the house that had been my home for the past nineteen years. It was the happiest moment in so many difficult months. Even little Honey came over to the wheelchair to let me pet her for just a minute.

The home health aide that an agency had provided was more than a disappointment. She mostly sat in a chair in the living room and watched TV. When I asked her to, she helped me to the bathroom, to the dining room for meals, to bed at night, and assisted me with a sponge bath and dressing in the morning. I had to call her several times during the night to get her to help me to the bedside commode. During the day, she was on either the phone or watching TV and did not offer to help Judy with meal preparation or any of the housework. She did not seem to like the pets and told them to get off my bed. I was glad to see her go and hoped she would never be back. The agency was sending out a replacement.

After she left, I tried to get up out of the bed on my own, but my left leg just would not function. I fell to the floor and called to Judy, who was in the next room. The paramedics came quickly and lifted me back into bed. They checked me over and said that I was OK. Judy told the home health aide that came to the house that afternoon that I had fallen. The aide said that she was required to report the incident to my attending physician. The nurse practitioner from Dr. Gates's office called and told us to be in her office the following morning.

The next day she came into the treatment room where we were sitting. I heard Judy ask, "Do I need to get my attorney?" She seemed to be much friendlier after that remark and explained that this was routine procedure following a fall in the home. She told us that she had arranged for me to go back to the skilled nursing facility, but I would be on the custodial side of the facility with no therapy for the next ten days. She maintained that this arrangement was consistent with Medicare regulations. I would be reevaluated in ten days to determine future placement. I was devastated.

I shared a room with a woman who had been in the facility for over twelve years. She had a huge collection of stuffed animals that took up about one-fourth of the small room. There was barely enough space for my bed and a small bedside stand on which a lamp with a low wattage bulb had been placed. The curtains in the room had to be drawn closed all of the time because of my roommate's visual problems. So I was crammed into a suffocating small space, in a dark room, in a narrow bed, with a lamp that did not emit enough light for me to read, and dreading mealtime that I shared with individuals who drooled with each bite of food. How could I live through ten days under these deplorable conditions?

Thank goodness for Judy's daily visits. We escaped out of the prison-like room into a corridor filled with individuals in wheelchairs who stared into space or napped with their heads hanging down on their chests. Others sat in their wheelchairs and watched TV hour after hour. There was moaning and groaning from some of the individuals as we passed by in a wheelchair on the way up to the unoccupied lobby. Would I be like that someday? On the other hand, even more frightening, how long will it be before I join these hopeless, helpless individuals?

After ten days, I was discharged back home with around-the-clock assistance and supervision, indefinitely. Home never felt so good. I promised Judy that I would never try to get out of the wheelchair or bed without assistance. Through a network of friends, Judy had secured the services of an LPN to live with us for the next four weeks.

Martha was a miracle worker and set about the task of my care with a very positive attitude. She knew what I needed but did not allow me to carry out any activities without her supervision and/or assistance. Besides all of these qualities, Martha made my miserable life fun.

In addition to Martha's full-time services, Judy had also arranged for the provision of home health services. An intake nurse visited me within two hours of my arrival home and arranged for me to restart therapy.

A physical therapist and an occupational therapist came to the house twice a week. The intake nurse made it very clear that I was never to try doing things on my own. I was to get assistance before attempting any activity. Martha nodded her head in agreement.

My condition improved almost miraculously during the four weeks that Martha spent with me. The physical therapist, a strong, muscular young man, walked me up

and down the stairs in the house (good leg first going up
and bad leg first coming down), up and down the long
driveway, and around the stone walk in the front yard.
He held me snug against his side with the gait belt for
balance and told me to concentrate on what I was doing.
I regained some confidence in my ability to ambulate
with a tripod cane, at least around the house, and always
with assistance and supervision. The occupational therapist worked with my left arm that continued to not function. It remained inert as it drooped down by my side or
outside the wheelchair. I had to be reminded to pick it
up and put it in my lap. She explained that my balance
would always be a problem if I did not sit straight in the
wheelchair and keep my left arm close by my side. Judy
and Martha joined me at the dining-room table as the
occupational therapist conducted the sessions on therapeutic exercise for my arm and balance.

After Martha's departure, home health aides came to
the house and stayed overnight. Along with assisting me
to the bedside commode during the night, they assisted
me with toileting, bathing, and getting dressed in the
early morning. Judy took me to outpatient physical therapy one hour a day, three days a week. Home health aides
came to the house during the day two days a week so that
Judy could grocery shop and do other chores.

Everything was progressing well until I fell in the
kitchen late one afternoon after we had come home from
physical therapy. My left leg just gave out. Judy called

9-1-1, and the paramedics came immediately. After ascertaining that I had no fractures, they said that I needed to go to the emergency room because my blood pressure was quite high. I had been home for over two months, and I detested the idea of leaving again for yet another hospital stay.

I was hospitalized late that evening so that my cardiologist could see me early the next day. After evaluating me, he arranged for me to have a pacemaker inserted the following afternoon. The surgical procedure went very smoothly, and the cardiologist assured me that I would be going home in twenty-four hours. My niece Tammy flew in from Chicago to relieve Judy, who had arranged a short respite visit with relatives in Texas.

I was discharged from the hospital on the afternoon that Judy left. Tammy seemed quite comfortable with helping me after the home health aide showed her how to assist me with ambulating and with routine daily activities. It was so good to be home again!

I had been home less than forty-eight hours when severe diarrhea started. I spent most of the evening on the bedside commode. Early the next morning, the home health aide told Tammy to call for an ambulance. I felt so badly for Tammy, who had thought that she was coming for a nice visit. She had found me in the hospital following surgery, had brought me home following my discharge, and now was having to provide full-time care to me. She stayed with me in the emergency room for several hours until I was readmitted to the hospital.

I was diagnosed with severe, acute diarrhea from bacteria of undetermined origin. I had contracted the virulent bacteria when I was hospitalized for the pacemaker insert. After administering massive doses of intravenous antibiotics, Dr. Gates arranged for me to return to the rehab side of the skilled nursing facility.

Tammy left the next day to return home. She accepted my sincere apologies for having put her through such a miserable ordeal, and we said our tearful good-byes.

It was back to the skilled nursing facility for more physical therapy and occupational therapy. There had been a change of staff so that I did not know them and they did not know me. Therefore, in addition to my new problems, I had to deal with new personnel. I was so weak from the bacterial episode that I could hardly walk. My appetite was poor, and I hated to go to the dining room, so I skipped most meals. I slowly and laboriously dressed myself in the morning and undressed in the evening. The previous exhilarating drills in physical therapy became a chore that I had to endure. The occupational therapist had little patience with my inability to perform daily routine activities. The nursing staff grew weary of my constant requests to be taken to the bathroom. Urinary urgency kept me awake at night. I was miserable and felt trapped in an unknown space in which there was no escape.

I grew much weaker during the five weeks back at the skilled nursing facility. I did not feel any real motivation to keep on trying. Everything seemed hopeless, and I felt helpless. I just wanted to go home.

Then an overwhelming and additional blow to my ego occurred during a conference Judy and I were asked to attend. After minimal deliberations, I heard the outcome of their collective decision: "You are not motivated to participate in the expected rehab activities. It is our best judgment that you be discharged to an assisted-living facility of your choice. The social worker will assist you in selecting a facility, if you so desire. You will be discharged in one week."

I looked at Judy's grim face and knew that she was having difficulty fathoming what had just transpired. The social worker went with us to my room and gave Judy the names of several reputable facilities in the nearby area.

Suddenly the space in my world was retracting, and there was no escape. I could almost feel the encumbering tugs to succumb to an increasing darkness. *What is going to happen to me? Where will I go next? Why is this happening to me? Is there no force or no being that can help me out of this encroaching darkness? How can I get out of this entrapment, this shrinking corner? I do not think I have the will to fight any longer.*

After considerable searching, Judy found an assisted-living facility that met each of the quality-of-care criteria that she had developed. I felt secure and comfortable in my bright, cheery, private room and was very impressed with Stephen and Helen, who were the owners and caregivers at Reed's Road. During meals in the attractive dining room, I sat at the head of the table with three individuals who also were residents at Reed's Road. Only one of the other patients was able to carry on a conversation with me.

Another drastic blow to my already deflated ego occurred when Judy and I met with Dr. Gates in his office a few days later. "You need to select a hospice service agency to provide the necessary care that you will need at Reed's Road. You have 'failure to thrive syndrome,' and hospice personnel will help you prepare for the next few weeks." What was I to do? I was not ready to die. I was so exhausted that my thoughts were almost incoherent. Back in the car, Judy took my hand and said, "We will get the help that is needed, and we will get through this somehow."

Under the instructions of Dr. Gates, I received numerous intramuscular injections of a strong antibiotic for a severe bladder infection and daily doses of a prescribed antidepressant. A physical therapist and a nurse from a hospice agency provided assistive care of bathing, dressing, and walking three times a week. Stephen and Helen encouraged me to eat small portions of food at each meal and to drink as much fluids as I could on an hourly basis. I remained in contact with reality through CNN TV. I watched the old Turner classics several times each day and tuned in to the morning and evening news. I read the local newspaper and tried to keep up with what was going on in Prescott. I phoned Judy several times each day, and she visited almost every day. I was unable to use the DVD that Grace had hooked up for me to watch movies. Friends dropped by for short visits. I was tucked into bed at about 8:00 p.m. and was awakened by Stephen at 7:00 a.m. I enjoyed conversing with five-year-old Anthony, son of Stephen and Helen. I had short conversations, at mealtime, with Susan, who had been a resident at Reed's Road for over four years. My niece Tammy called me often and encouraged me to keep fighting. In short, I kept myself busy during those first few weeks at the assisted-living facility, and I tried not to think of what Dr. Gates had told me about "failure to thrive."

It seemed that a miracle had occurred when I next visited Dr. Gates in his office. He was astounded with the progress that I had made, particularly in ambulating. I had gained nine pounds. I spoke more distinctly. He ordered continuation of antibiotics orally, continuation of antidepressants, and physical therapy at an outpatient facility for the next six weeks. I was thankful when he assured me that I no longer needed hospice-care services.

By the end of summer (after three months at Reed's Road), I felt well enough to go for a short stay at a resort in nearby Sedona. After securing Dr. Gates's permission, Judy and a friend, Margaret, arranged for a couple of overnights at a large cabin located in an incredibly beautiful, secluded setting beside a creek in which the water flowed gently over the rocks. The tranquility soothed my soul. I felt a renewed commitment to try to get my body functioning better so that I could go home again.

The days that followed our relaxing expedition were filled with numerous activities. I employed Caroline to assist me in walking for thirty to forty-five minutes three times a week. Dr. Gates ordered physical therapy for my left arm and hand twice a week for six weeks. I practiced the range-of-motion exercises back in my room on the days I did not go to therapy. I kept abreast of current events by watching TV, reading the local newspaper daily, and reading *Time* magazine weekly. I enjoyed short conversations with Susan during meals. I learned a great deal about Legos and small birdhouses from Anthony, who had started preschool. He shared his creative imagination with me, particularly during dinner. In return, I helped him with his homework.

Judy took me to the movies almost every week, where I enjoyed popcorn and Diet Pepsi. I particularly enjoyed my Sunday visits at home with Judy, Rosie, and Honey. Caroline usually joined us for the special brunch that Judy had prepared, and she helped me to the bathroom. I welcomed the visits from friends and previous neighbors who shared news of what was occurring in the community.

I was fitted with a hearing aide that never seemed to help my hearing. Bladder infections persisted, which necessitated a visit to Dr. Gates's office every four weeks. After each visit, antibiotics were prescribed for ten days. Either Judy or Caroline took me to follow-up visits with my cardiologist every three months and to an ophthalmologist every six months. Caroline took me to a hairdresser every six weeks. I was busy!

Stephen and I carried on lively discussions and conversations as he assisted me daily with routine activities, with ambulating to the dining room for meals, and with frequent trips to the bathroom. I steadily gained weight with the good meals that Helen prepared. I relished a small glass of wine with dinner each evening. Stephen and Helen were meeting most of my physical needs. In addition, I enjoyed their company.

As the seasons transitioned through the next year, I felt changes in Judy's behavior. We seemed to have little understanding or empathy toward each other, and we were unable to share our feelings with each other. Sometimes we were short with each other, and our daily conversations were usually unsympathetic. After some intense reflection, I realized that I had been harboring intense feelings of guilt for having a stroke and for being disabled the past two years. I felt that I had deprived Judy of a normal life since the stroke. She had been involved constantly in making decisions regarding my care. She had dealt with numerous facility selections, with renovations in our home, with numerous strangers that came into our house to assist with my care, and with my personal and business affairs as my power of attorney. She had no time for herself. The stress of all these and other continuous responsibilities was taking a toll on her and on our relationship. I was unable to alter the situation other than to succumb to my mounting feelings of guilt. Where would I go from here? I would not be able to drive safely again, neither could I be physically active and take long trips as I did before my stroke. Additionally, there was the possibility of having another stroke and a continuation of the need for 24-7 assisted care. I was so tired of having to adjust constantly to new environments and new people. My options were extremely limited.

I realized that I needed to connect with my new self that was emerging from the trauma that had been imposed on me from the stroke. Almost all of the rehab and restorative activities had been directed toward improving and maintaining my physical functioning, particularly my left side that had been affected by the stroke. Slowly, I began to understand that my body would never be the same as it was three years before. I did not know what the future held for me. The past was gone, and the future was unknown. I, like all other living human beings, had only the present to grow anew and to become complete and whole again. What a difficult lesson to learn!

With these new awakenings of self, Judy's decision to sell my car did not hurl me back into oblivion. I could buy another car when and if I was able to drive again. However, when she told me that she thought it was time to sell our house that we co-owned and move to a smaller one, I panicked. Where would I live? Judy assured me that I would always have a home as long as she lived. She said that it was a matter of changing addresses and down-sizing to our decreasing needs for space.

I liked the small house that she purchased, but she had made one of the two bedrooms into a study. I wondered where an assistant would stay when I came home. The closet in the study contained all of my clothes that I had accumulated through the years. I insisted that she keep them, even though I had not worn most of them for three or four years. Perhaps I would wear them someday.

Judy had done a nice job decorating the house and having grab bars added in one of the bathrooms for me. My comfortable rising recliner beckoned me to have a seat each time I went for a visit.

Rosie did not adjust well to being confined in the smaller space at the new house. I was miserable when Judy suggested that we give her up for adoption. I agreed with Judy that she needed more space so that she could run and take long walks. I realized that Judy was not able to walk her because of her painful back. I remember sitting on my bed at the care center the night after Rosie had left for her new adoptive home. I looked over at the picture of my dog that was in a frame on the dresser and softly said, "I am so sorry, Rosie, that I am not there to take care of you." Again, I was apologizing and feeling guilty because I could not fulfill the expectations of others due to the stroke.

It was like an epiphany when I realized that I could not entirely blame the stroke for everything that happened over the last three tumultuous years of my life. I was entrapped by guilt, and I felt compelled to apologize constantly to my caregivers and to Judy. I decided that counseling could help me deal with the negative feelings that were keeping me from recovering from the ravaging effects of the stroke. Thankfully, Rosie did not reply when I told her, "I am sorry that I cannot take care of you."

Along with all of these changes that were occurring in my outside life, I kept falling. The most recent of my twenty-four falls was the only one that caused serious repercussions. I was at home with Judy, and she was assisting me in moving from a dining-room chair to the recliner in the living room. I was engrossed with a golf game on TV and did not follow Judy's instructions (orders) to move closer to the recliner. I attempted to sit down before I reached the recliner, and I fell flat on my back and left side. An X-ray indicted a hairline fracture of the humerus. An ice cap during the night alleviated the pain, to some degree. Range-of-motion exercises with a physical therapist helped me return to normal functioning within a few weeks.

Almost four years have gone by since that fatal day that changed my life so drastically. I have to keep reminding myself daily that the past is gone, the future is unknown, and I only have the present to deal with the changes that have occurred in my life. These selected passages from Lindbergh's *Gift from the Sea* have assisted me in facing challenges that I encounter each day. "I am looking at... the outside of my life—the shell. The final answer, however...is always inside. One is free, like the hermit crab, to change one's shell." Nevertheless, the inside remains constant.

My outside shell has changed, but I still love life. I still love my family and friends, and I enjoy talking with them about current events. I am grateful that my mental faculties are functioning so that I can keep abreast of what is happening on this planet. I appreciate tremendously the daily assistance provided by Stephen and Helen. I am thankful for the constant devotion and attention that Judy has provided. My steps may falter, but my essence persists.

Ann Morrow Lindbergh, *Gift from the Sea* (New York: Pantheon Books, 2005), p. 29.

Four

ENTRAPMENT: BECOMING A CAREGIVER – JUANITA MURPHY

I awakened from a sound sleep and jumped out of bed in one quick movement. I had an overwhelming feeling that something was desperately wrong. It was a few minutes past 7:00 a.m., and Maria was not making her usual noises with early morning chores. She was supposed to get up at 6:30 a.m. to get ready for the house cleaner, who was arriving at 8:30 a.m. She had set the radio alarm in the bedroom next door. Where was Maria, and what was she doing?

I hurriedly searched the living room, but I did not see Maria. A radio was playing loudly in her bedroom, and the bedside lamp was on. Maybe she was still asleep. As I entered the bedroom, I saw Maria lying on her back in the middle of the bed. Her pillow was askew, and the cover sheet was rumpled in a mass. Her left leg was bent under her body, and her eyes were closed. Gurgling noises were coming from her open mouth.

I called, "Maria!" She did not open her eyes.

"Maria, Maria, wake up! Can you hear me? Say something, Maria!"

I turned the radio off and reached over and touched Maria's left arm. Her eyes remained closed. The gurgling noises continued. Her breathing seemed shallow. I lifted Maria's left hand. There was no response.

"Maria, can you squeeze my hand?" Still no response.

"Can you turn your face toward me?" No response. The gurgling noises seemed to be getting louder. "Can you hear me?"

"Maria, I think that you have had a stroke. I am going to get the emergency personnel out here right now." There was no movement, just the continuous, irregular gurgling sounds from her throat.

With shaking fingers that seemed to have lost their functioning, I dialed 911 from the bedside phone. I was almost hysterical as I described Maria's condition to the person who answered the phone. The receptionist was asking too many questions and taking too much precious time. I nervously repeated the directions to the house. "Please, please just get over here!"

I tried to turn Maria onto her right side with the hope that she could breathe more easily, but I was not able to move the dead weight. I reached for Maria's right wrist to check her pulse. It seemed to be very rapid and irregular.

I kept calling her name and told her that the paramedics were coming to help her. I kept wondering what else I could do until they got there. No answers came.

Should I change out of my nightgown, or stay with her? I reluctantly left Maria's side and ran back into my bedroom to change into a blouse, pants, and shoes. *What should I wear? What will I be doing today? Hurry! Hurry! Get back in there to see about Maria!*

The zipper on my pants did not seem to close. I fumbled with the buttons on the blouse and slipped my feet into shoes. I hurriedly washed my face, brushed my hair, and ran back in to check on Maria. Rosie, the dog, was up on the bed with Maria. She was using her paw to try to arouse Maria and looking into her face as if to awaken her. Honey, the cat, was curled up on the pillow near Maria's head. The gurgling sound from Maria's throat continued, and her eyes remained closed. She did not seem to be aware of the bright light from the bedroom light.

"Where are those paramedics? They are just up the road. Have they lost their way? What's taking so long? Please, please help me!"

After what seemed to be hours, the emergency medical technicians arrived with the siren blaring and the red light flashing. They parked the fire engine at the end of the long driveway, and two men loaded with a stretcher and other emergency equipment ran up to the house. I was standing on the front porch and assured them that this was the right address. They ran through the front room door, and I led them to the bedroom where Maria was lying unconscious.

They immediately checked her breathing, pulse, and blood pressure. One paramedic put a pillow under her head to assist her breathing. The other paramedic checked her arms and legs and said, "She does not seem to have any feeling on her left side."

I told them that I thought that she had a stroke and that she had a transient ischemic attack about five months ago, had been hospitalized, and had recovered with no apparent ill effect. One of the men asked what medications she was taking. I ran into the kitchen and opened the pantry door. The medication list that I had just revised one month ago was pinned to the door. After the transient ischemic attack, Maria and I both knew the importance of having a copy of the list available at all times. I hurried back into the bedroom and gave the list to the nearest paramedic.

They asked me to take the dog and cat into another part of the house, because the dog did not seem to want them touching her mom. After removing them, I heard one of the men on the phone saying, "...and make it quick. You will see our engine parked at the head of the driveway. Just drive on up to the house. Come in through the front door. Hurry."

My hopes that this was not serious came crashing to the ground. I looked at Maria lying so motionless on the bed and noticed that the left side of her face was droop-ing. Another bad sign. She squeezed my hand with her right hand when I asked her to. A hopeful sign. She was able to open her eyes, but the left one drooped. She seemed to recognize me as her eyelids fluttered from the bright light. She tried to speak, but only throaty sounds came out. Not a good sign.

The emergency ambulance arrived in a few minutes. One of the paramedics ran out to help the ambulance personnel with the collapsed wheeled gurney. After some conferring, they decided that it would be impos-sible to bring Maria through the narrow doorway of the bedroom if the wheels were extended. The three men carefully moved her onto the flattened stretcher, placed her on her back with a pillow under her head, and strapped her on the stretcher. They laboriously moved her into the living room. I gave the ambulance driver Maria's drivers license as identification and told him that her updated medical insurance information was on file at the hospital.

In the meantime, Patsy, the housekeeper, had arrived at the appointed time of 8:30 a.m. She left her car parked at the end of the driveway. I went out on the front porch and asked her to pull her car out on the street so that the ambulance could exit.

As she came up the driveway after parking her car, she started yelling, "What is going on here? Is something wrong with Maria or you? I followed an ambulance for a while, and then they turned into here. Tell me, what is happening?"

Her state of panic only added to the confusion of moving Maria out to the ambulance. She went over to the gurney and said, "Maria, has there been an accident? Are you OK? What happened? Just talk to me."

Maria's eyes fluttered open briefly as she looked up from the stretcher. An inaudible sound came from her throat.

Maria was carried out of our home, down the steep front steps, and into the waiting ambulance. They started the trip to the emergency room with the siren shrieking and red lights flaring in the quiet neighborhood. I had told the driver that I would meet them in the emergency room in a few minutes. I had not even said good-bye to Maria. I wondered if she would be alive when I saw her next. I could not grasp the vast changes that would alter the remainder of my life. I was totally unable to comprehend the magnitude of what had occurred in the last two hours.

I slowly walked back inside with Patsy and looked at a house that had only recently been a lovely and loving home. It did not look or feel the same. I was brought back to sudden reality by Patsy's continuous demands to tell her what had happened. I related the series of events to her as I prepared the morning meals for Rosie and Honey.

My usual breakfast of coffee, toast, orange juice, and milk was tasteless. But I consumed it, since I did not know when I would be eating again. I asked Patsy to stay the allotted time of six hours and to watch after the pets. I wrote out a check for her services and told her that I would be calling her here as soon as I knew more about Maria's condition. With Maria's purse on one arm, and my purse (with the cell phone) on the other arm, I started the slow journey of seven miles to the hospital emergency room.

As I was driving down the familiar route to my destination, I tried to stay within the speed limit and look only straight ahead. I went over the events of the previous evening, when Maria had told me she was setting the alarm so she could get up early and I could sleep in. She had not complained of anything unusual, and she had taken her prescribed medications compliantly. When had her stroke occurred? Had she tried to call me? Did she realize what had happened? All of these thoughts raced through my mind as I headed toward the unknown.

I was quite familiar with the entrance and setup of the emergency room, since I had been there on numerous occasions previously with Maria. The receptionist asked me to go over to the admitting clerk and provide needed information so that they could get Maria admitted. I told her that I needed to see Maria first and that I would come out after I had seen her to complete the transaction. She reluctantly called an escort to take me to the cubicle in which they had placed Maria.

Maria was lying on her back with the head of the gurney elevated. Oxygen was flowing from one tube, and IV fluids were flowing from another tube, into her arm. A nurse and a technician were hooking her up to heart-monitoring machine. They explained to Maria what they were doing with each procedure. I went over to her side, and she opened her right eye and said, "Hi," in a garbled tone. I took her hand, told her where she was, and asked if a doctor had been in yet to see her. The nurse quickly explained that a doctor had examined her almost immediately upon arrival. Blood had been drawn, and she would be going to the imagery center shortly, after they had her vital signs stabilized.

I called my nurse friend, Angie, and told her what had happened. She said she would be there shortly. The next few hours seemed a cognitive blur. The doctor came in and told us that Maria had suffered a massive stroke, and that it was probably a hemorrhagic occurrence on the right side of her brain, which affected her left side. He explained that there was obvious left-side paralysis of the face, arm, leg, and, indeed, the entire side of the body. The loss of consciousness just following the stroke was usual and would subside with time. She would have slurred speech, aphasia, blurred vision, impaired breathing and swallowing, and altered coordination for an inestimable amount of time. His plan of action was to have comprehensive lab works and cerebral imagery completed to determine the severity of the damage to the brain. In the meantime, he assured us that they would do everything possible to stabilize her condition before admitting her to the hospital.

The next five hours were a blur. Maria was wheeled out of the cubicle to the imagery center with all the lines attached. She looked at me when she left, and I thought I saw a smile. When she returned, I found that she had urinated involuntarily. Linens for the gurney were changed. She seemed to be saying a few words that were not coherent. Angie talked with her soothingly and told her she would be all right. Again, I thought I saw a smile.

Her primary care physician, Dr. Gates, came into the cubicle and talked with us during his lunch break. He confirmed her diagnosis of a severe hemorrhagic stroke, and he told us that Maria was going to be admitted to the hospital as soon as a bed became available. He told us that he had written orders for Maria to be evaluated by a physical therapist, an occupational therapist, and a speech therapist either late that evening or early the next morning. Dr. Gates carefully explained that these evaluations were necessary to ascertain her rehabilitation potential. He commented to me, "The next seventy-two hours are critical, and we will do everything possible to restore as many bodily functions as we can. It is a matter of time, the severity and extent of the hemorrhage, and her endurance." He left with a handshake and remarked, "Hang in there."

Angie went to the hospital cafeteria and brought me back a sandwich. The nurse put an ice cube in Maria's mouth, but she immediately started strangling. I was getting the feeling that Maria had been undone in some basic manner.

Then came some good news. They would be moving Maria upstairs to a patient's room at 3:00 p.m. She had been in the emergency room for the past six hours. During that time, she had regained consciousness, uttered a few audible words, and swallowed a few ice chips with extreme difficulty. Her vital signs had become more stable. These positive signs gave me hope that she was not going to die.

The move upstairs to her assigned room was carefully orchestrated by several nurses and an orderly. Even though cardiac monitoring was ceased temporarily, they were able to continue dispersing oxygen through a nasal tube, and the intravenous tubes were guarded during the ride up an elevator and into a room. The real test was how to get her off the gurney and onto the hospital bed without interruption. I heard a loud, "Mission accomplished!" from inside the room. One of the nurses suggested that I go in to see Maria for a minute or two and then go home. "You both need some rest. You can call the nurses' station at any time to inquire about her condition." I left reluctantly after telling Maria that I was leaving but would be calling frequently. She squeezed my hand with her right hand and said, "OK." At least she knew me and was forming words.

I drove home slowly with continuous thoughts of how the day had unwound. I knew that I had to pull myself together to take care of the pets and the house. What a fantastic wonder Patsy had been! She had cleaned the house thoroughly, including washing Maria's bedclothes. She had made the beds and left folded linens on the washer. She left me a note to call her when I returned home.

I took care of Rosie and Honey first, as usual. Rosie had jumped upon my legs when I walked into the house from the garage. I told her that her mom was very sick but would be coming home soon. After taking care of the pets, I just wandered around the house and tried to put the horrible events of the day into some kind of perspective. I did not have a clue about what to expect for the next twenty-four hours.

In response to my phone call a few hours later, the nurse related, "Maria is sleeping now. She took a few sips of soup for dinner, but she was not able to swallow. We are giving her 'thickened water,' and she swallowed a couple of sips. We put in a retention catheter because of her urinary incontinence. She is getting continuous intravenous fluids with a lot of essential medications added. Her vitals are stable, and she is resting. I will call you if there are changes."

I went out onto the back patio and gazed up at the starry sky. *Why us, God? What do you want from me?* Maria had undergone two low-risk heart ablations and two high-risk complex intestinal surgeries within the past three years. Her attending surgeon had given her a 40 percent chance of survival from the first intestinal procedure. She had survived and was enjoying a reprieve from the intense medical care. She had followed the cardiologist's prescriptions precisely. Following the transient ischemic attack just five months ago, we had flown to Maui for my birthday and stayed at a lush, ocean-side resort. Just three weeks ago, we had flown to Texas and Oklahoma to visit with my family. We both had enjoyed the two trips immensely, even though I was able to ambulate for only short distances because of acute pain in my back. Life had seemed so good just three weeks ago. Traveling had been among our greatest pleasures since retirement.

I was unable to stop the torrent of tears that had been welling up all day. Why? Why? No answers were forthcoming. After a hastily prepared dinner, the pets and I went into the bedroom to make a last call to the nurses' station. They reported, "She is about the same, and she has asked for water for her dry mouth. She swallows the thickened water with difficulty." I hung up and tried to get some sleep. I slept fitfully and kept seeing Maria's drooping face in my dreams.

Dr. Gates called me early the next morning and told me that Maria's condition had improved during the night. Her speech was more understandable and lucid. She would be going down to imagery to evaluate the hemorrhagic site and extent of the stroke. The therapists would begin their evaluations during the day. He encouraged me to stay at home and get some rest. "We will let you know if there are any negative changes. She seems to be out of the woods now. The next seventy-two hours are critical. If the bleeding has stopped, and if the evaluations from the therapists indicate that her rehabilitation potential is good enough, we will be sending her to the rehab hospital. Right now she is stabilized."

I tried to busy myself with the usual early morning chores, but I could not concentrate or complete a task. After calling the nurses' station two times, I felt an urgency to see for myself that she was sitting up on the side of the bed with assistance. She had reclined by the time I arrived in her hospital room, but she waved her right hand at me when I stepped to her bedside. Tears coursed uncontrollably down my cheeks as I took her hand and gazed at her lopsided smile. Janice, Maria's nurse for the day, told me that two of the therapists had been in to perform an initial evaluation. The third would be in later in the day and again the next day. Janice explained about the need to give Maria small amounts of thickened water, since her ability to swallow had been affected, and she choked on plain water. Maria would be on a liquid diet indefinitely.

Soon Maria was sleeping soundly, and she only roused when Janice came in to attend to her needs. Janice promised me that she would call me when she went off duty at 7:00 p.m. Maria uttered a weak "good-bye" as I left. Dr. Gates phoned me that evening to let me know that the brain hemorrhage seemed to have subsided and that the therapists' evaluation looked somewhat promising. I was receiving phone calls every few minutes from friends and family. My response was guarded, since I did not have answers to most of their numerous questions.

After another sleepless night filled with a thousand questions but no answers, I tried to develop a plan for the day, including how to take care of the phone calls. Dr. Gates called to let me know that Maria had an uneventful night and that they were going to do repeat imagery to make sure everything was OK with her brain. He closed with, "She is really going to need your help now." And thus, the day began.

I was able to discern very slight improvements in her speech when I visited that afternoon. Janice said that she had swallowed some cooked cereal for breakfast and some thick broth for lunch. She indicated that they were adding special medications to her continuous intravenous solutions. She had spent most of her working day with Maria, and she would be Maria's nurse again the next day. The therapists had been in for their second day of evaluations.

Janice's devotion to caring for Maria was so obvious. Dr. Gates's message that evening was, "Everything seems to be looking better. Tomorrow we will have a more

definitive plan. We need a little more confirming data."
The contact plan that I had worked out involved one
person communicating with several other people, and it
was working fairly well. I sent the lead person a progress
report and fell into bed with the pets.

Janice called me at about 8:00 a.m. and told me that
Maria had a good night and was asking for me. Janice
said, "Don't rush down here. I think that she is aware that
she is in the hospital. See you later."

When I arrived at the hospital a few hours later,
Maria was sitting on the edge of the bed while the physical therapist conducted an examination. She emitted
a fairly audible, "Good morning," and raised her right
hand in a greeting. Janice came in to feed her lunch of
thickened orange juice and broth. Maria seemed to have
difficulty with the food that was placed in her mouth,
but she was able to swallow small amounts of liquids
without gagging. Janice told me that Maria's blood work
from the morning indicated that almost everything was
outside normal limits. They were doing a final cranial
scan that afternoon, and Dr. Gates had been in contact
with the rehab hospital. Janice patiently answered my
questions of when, why, where, how she was going to
get there, and what could I do in the interim. She told
me that there were no open beds today at the rehab
hospital, but with projected discharges, there would be
a few beds available over the weekend, which began the
next day.

Dr. Gates gave me much the same news when he called me that evening. Maria would be going by ambulance to the rehab hospital the following afternoon. This was great news! Her functioning could improve with concentrated rehabilitation efforts. Again he stated, "She is going to need your help." I called my phone contact to relate the new developments. My mind kept searching for answers as to why this was happening. I tried to comprehend the magnitude of the rapid series of events that had foreclosed reality for these last few days.

Maria was admitted to a semiprivate room, in which the other bed was occupied. She tolerated but grew weary of the lengthy intake sessions with an admissions clerk, a social worker, and a physician. She gave affirmative or negative monosyllabic responses to their questions. A nurse oriented her to the call signal and told her that dinner would be served at 5:00 p.m. She gave me a list of personal items, things I would need to bring in for Maria, and told me that I would be responsible for laundering Maria's clothing.

The rehab physician in charge of her care told us that Medicare allowed only twenty-one days for the intensive rehabilitative care that Maria was going to require. Physical therapists would be working on her range of motion, muscular strengthening, and coordination. Occupational therapists would be working on self-care activities such as grooming, dressing, bathing, and toileting. Speech therapists would be working on her oropharyngeal dysphasia, which included swallowing problems, speech changes, and left-side facial drooping. The ultimate goal was to maximize her functional ability and increase her independence. She would be in therapy for at least three hours each day for five days a week for the next three weeks. He added that I was welcome to visit at any time, but my presence might be distracting during therapy sessions.

Maria looked so frail and helpless lying in the hospital bed. We both started crying. I tried to console her with assurances. "We are going to get through this. It may take some time, but you are going to be OK." She just shook her head. I told her that I would see her the next day, and that Rosie and Honey missed her, but they were OK.

I made the much-longer round trip of thirty miles to the rehab hospital almost every day during the next three weeks. One of the therapists related the difficulty of getting Maria involved with her therapy because she was so easily distracted and could not concentrate. They had to keep reminding her to focus on the task at hand. One therapist said she thought that Maria did not realize the gravity of her situation. Her problem-solving ability was markedly absent. Her balance needed constant attention because she pushed to the left. She had extreme difficulty following commands when transferring from one surface to another. She ate very slowly, primarily due to attention deficits. She did not seem to comprehend their directions about fall precautions and safe mobility. Maria reported to me each day that she was absolutely exhausted and just wanted to get into bed. She just wanted out of that wheelchair. She really detested having a roommate and having to go down to the cafeteria, in the wheelchair, for all of her meals.

After the first week of intensive therapy, the reports indicated some slight improvement. Her speech was more intelligible, and she was forming sentences. She was eating blended food and meat and drinking thin liquids without gagging. I made arrangements with our friends, Grace and Katrina, to bring Maria's dog Rosie to visit her on Sunday. Rosie ran to Maria and jumped up into her lap when she came out of the hospital door in the wheelchair. Grace helped Maria with calming Rosie down and took Rosie for short walks while Maria watched. Both friends remarked at how good Maria looked and how much better she was than the previous week. Rosie's visit with Maria the following Sunday went much better. The dog was not so hyperactive, and Maria was able to hold Rosie in her lap for some of the time.

I made several visits to see Maria in the early evenings so that I could have dinner with her in the cafeteria. She went over the day's activities and told me what she was doing in each of the therapy sessions. She told me she hated the food because, "They just pour it all in a blender, and you can't tell the eggs from the sausage or pancakes." It took her over an hour to consume the small portions. Later, I asked that she be assigned a seat facing the wall so that she would not be so easily distracted by others in the room while eating.

The social worker's office was just across the hall from Maria's room. She came in several times while I was there just to check on how things were going. At the beginning of the third week of Maria's hospital stay, the social worker came in to tell us that a discharge-planning conference would be held on a particular day that week. I responded that I would not be able to attend because I had a doctor's appointment in Phoenix on that date. She said that they would change it to the next day so I could attend, and then she gave me the names of three reputable skilled nursing facilities in the area from which to choose. I followed the social worker back to her office, and she told me that two of the places did not have vacancies at the time. I told her that the remaining facility had a poor reputation with regard to patient care. A close friend had been there and had asked to be moved because of lack of care.

I was on the way to the specialist's office in Phoenix when I received a call on my cell phone from Maria's niece, Tammy, who lived outside of Chicago. She told me that I had not called her over the weekend, and she was worried about Aunt Maria. After assuring Tammy that Maria was improving gradually and apprising her of the forthcoming move to a skilled nursing facility, I told her where I was and why I was going to Phoenix. She apologized. I had hoped that I would have a few hours reprieve from the constant ringing of the phone.

After visiting with the specialist, he arranged for me to return in two weeks for neurological surgery on my chronically underactive bladder. He told me that a hospital in Phoenix would be calling me within the next two weeks regarding the date and time of admission for the outpatient surgery. Another rung was added to my ladder of growing despair. How could I escape from the continuous barrage of overwhelming episodes that had been going on in my life for almost a month? I was unable to identify any feasible answers as I drove back home. I felt engulfed in a whirlpool from which there were no exits.

At home that evening, I went out on the patio with the pets and let the pent-up tears drain from my soul. A haze of depression engulfed me. Deep-seated sobs from the pits of my body left me grasping for air. *Death* and *dying*—those unutterable words kept slipping through my mind. It seemed that my only alternative was to succumb to a safe haven of denial regarding the severity and prognosis of Maria's condition.

I was abruptly thrust back into reality by a phone call from the social worker apprising me of the discharge meeting the next morning. After a dismal, tasteless dinner of leftovers that a neighbor had kindly brought, I sent an e-mail detailing what had happened to Maria and her subsequent hospitalizations. I let the e-mail recipients know that she would be moving to a local skilled nursing facility in the next few days. I thanked them for their loving thoughts and prayers, and for the flowers, plants, and get-well cards that they had sent to Maria. Sleep enshrouded me as the pets and I fell into bed.

The therapists gave an account of their activities and of Maria's progress during the planning conference. The conference leader turned to Maria and asked which of the skilled nursing facilities she had decided to move into following discharge. I was absolutely astounded to hear Maria submit the name of the facility that the social worker and I had crossed off the list because of its poor reputation. When I objected, the conference leader said, "It is Maria's decision. Group dismissed."

Back in Maria's room, I confronted her with her decision and pointed out that we had decided against that particular facility when we discussed it. The social worker intervened, and I went across the hall with her. She apprised me that there were no vacancies in the facility that we had decided on before, but they were expecting a discharge the following day. She assured me that she would use her influence to get Maria admitted there when the discharge occurred. "Just go home and get some rest. You look worn out." I followed her advice. She called me that evening to let me know that Maria could be admitted to the desired facility the next day. I thanked her profusely.

The move to the skilled nursing facility was uneventful, and the admission process was lengthy but informative.

Thank goodness Maria had a private room that was bright and cheery with sunlight beaming through the windows. The admitting personnel told us that she would be eating in the dining room and would be seated at a specified place. Therapy sessions would start at 6:00 a.m. the following Monday and would be conducted five days a week. They would label her clothes and would take care of her personal laundry. Her medication list had been sent, along with other documents. Maria emitted her one-sided smile and thanked them for their kind attention. I was pleased with her newfound ability to carry on a meaningful conversation and to enunciate words so distinctly. I left her with a cell phone. I wrote our home phone number in large numbers on a piece of paper and taped the paper to her bedside stand. I hugged her closely and went back to the world of mundane survival activities—grocery shopping, house cleaning, opening mail, tending the pets, paying the bills, calling the starters on the phone-call tree, and doing the laundry.

Maria settled into the prescribed routine without too much difficulty. She called me once or twice a day on the cell phone, and I called her often. I visited her almost every day, and other friends dropped by for short visits, particularly over the weekends, when she was not involved with therapy. She was able to tolerate soft and chopped foods, but she still did not have a good appetite. She reluctantly became accustomed to the 6:00 a.m. sessions with the occupational therapist, who helped her with dressing, bathing, and grooming. Nursing assistants helped her with toileting after instructions and safety precautions from the occupational therapist. The physical therapists tried to teach her how to use the wheelchair without assistance, but that proved to be too difficult because she only had the use of her "good" hand. They spent considerable time talking with her about safety factors, particularly while ambulating and transferring from one surface to another. She continued to be easily distracted while receiving assistance from therapists.

One evening I received a phone call from the head nurse, informing me that Maria had fallen in the bathroom, but she seemed to be OK. I later learned that Maria had gone into the bathroom by herself, and as she was starting to sit, she lost her balance. She fell onto the toilet stool with such force that it broke the water pipe. Water was gushing everywhere. A plumber came to repair the damages, and housekeeping cleaned up the water mess. Maria was moved to another room. Fortunately, she did not sustain any bodily injuries. Her ego was badly bruised.

The skilled nursing facility encouraged visits from patients' pets, so Katrina, Grace, and I took Rosie in to see Maria on several Sundays. We met in a large activities room down the hall from Maria's room. After a rambunctious greeting, Rosie usually settled down beside Maria to be petted, or got into her lap.

It was difficult to leave Maria, but I went to Phoenix for my scheduled surgery. A friend, Mary, provided transportation for the overnight trip and stayed with me while the surgery was being conducted. I had high hopes that the electrical implant would bring my bladder back to normal. Even with the trauma of surgery, the twenty-four-hour reprieve from worrying about Maria was a stress reliever.

Unfortunately, the electrical implant did not alter the problem, so ten days later Mary and I made another overnight trip to Phoenix to have the implant surgically removed. The short reprieve did little to lessen the mounting stress and bitter depression that was beginning to consume my being. I realized that I was becoming increasingly unable to care for myself and had been unable to provide any physical care for Maria.

My limited ability to provide any physical care for Maria was largely due to the tremendous pain in my lower back region that I had almost continuously for the past three years. The cause of pain had been diagnosed as osteoarthritis and vertebral stenosis. Along with steroidal anti-inflammatory drugs, I had several rounds of physical therapy, both of which suppressed the symptoms and inflammation. I used a walking cane to assist with balance when I ambulated. When the pain became so intense that I could barely ambulate, I had epidural injections. These gave me almost immediate relief, but only for short periods of time. I had the injections every three months for two years. I was advised not to lift anything weighing more than eight pounds. I was not able to take Rosie for walks due to my restricted ability to ambulate safely. The vicious cycle continued: pain, stress, all-consuming anxiety, depression, and unrelenting fatigue. I did not know how much longer I could go on with the problems associated with both our physical and emotional helplessness. I had no one with whom I could discuss the depths of my plight, and I certainly could not share my feelings with Maria. Other than my niece, Denise, my family rarely asked about Maria when they called.

I felt trapped, or at least cornered to such a degree, that there was no feasible way out. With each new episode in either my life or in Maria's life, the burden weighed heavier. My only relief was our friends and our pets. My moments of despair were increasing and mounting in intensity.

In the meantime, Maria seemed to be settling into the expected routine at the skilled nursing facility. She looked forward to the Sunday visits from Rosie, and she adjudged the food as tolerable. She became more adept at using the cell phone, and she called me at home at least twice per day. I was her invited guest for Thanksgiving, and friends Betty and Angie were her invited guests for Christmas.

The chief occupational therapist at the skilled nursing facility came to the house in late December to inspect it for needed alterations before Maria's planned discharge the last week in January. The prescribed ramp for wheelchair entry was constructed and installed; grab bars were installed in the shower and next to the commode in the bathroom; a bedside commode and several packages of Depends were placed in the large bedroom; the height of the bed was lowered; and eighteen throw rugs and carpets were removed and hauled upstairs. The house took on the appearance of a residence for disabled occupants.

A call on New Year's Day from the head nurse at the skilled nursing facility indicating that Maria had taken a rather serious fall while trying to get into bed by herself threw me back into a state of panic. I immediately called Maria, and she told me that her left leg had just given way, and she fell hard behind her bed. She said that she had some pain in her back, left arm, and left leg, but she assured me that she was OK. The following day, the head nurse told me that Maria might have had another small stroke, so she had called Dr. Gates. A nurse practitioner from Dr. Gates's office came over late that afternoon and found that her blood pressure was exceedingly high. She ordered emergency medications to lower Maria's blood pressure and asked that Maria be on bed rest (except to use the bedside commode) for the next forty-eight hours. Passive range-of-motion exercises were ordered. How would this new incident alter Maria's planned discharge in a little over three weeks? "We will just have to wait and see."

"Just wait and see," indeed, after three months of sheer hell, including mounting stress, unbearable loneliness, constant demands to be one place and then another, continuous phone calls, and increasing requests for information from various insurance companies. That night I realized that I had moved from the grieving stage of denial to anger. I went out on the deck and screamed into a dark abyss, "Why, why, why?" Then the forbidden expression, "Goddamn," emerged from my soul. I said it repeatedly and added that I was Goddamn mad. I pounded the cushions of the lawn chairs with my fists and finally asked myself, "To whom or to what am I screaming?" Then it occurred to me that I was not only angry with all that was happening to Maria and me, but I was also angry with Maria. There it was. But how could that be? That was impossible. I loved Maria and needed her. I felt like a fool as shame and guilt invaded my being. Maria had no control over the past five years of four surgeries, numerous hospitalizations, and more recently the stroke. I cried out to the vast cosmic force that ruled the universe that I could not take it anymore. There were no answers. I struggled limply into bed and sobbed uncontrollably.

I started building a protective façade around me to deal with the constant bombardments of stress and demands. I hid my usual friendly demeanor beneath a guise of stern directness that bordered on harshness. Sometimes I found it difficult to carry on a conversation in which the mundane things of life were being discussed. I searched for help and found it among my friends. Grace developed an e-mail tree to send out frequent reports on

Maria's status, and she took Rosie for walks in the neighborhood. Others brought food for me and the pets. Mary assisted me in finding home health aides that I would need in the future. I retained my protective façade for the next two years and allowed penetrations only when the situation demanded a less stern approach.

Maria was back into her previous routine of therapies after the fall. Her previous level of function had been compromised during the few down days. Then the inevitable discharge conference was called. The occupational therapist reported that the house was ready for Maria's return. She would need constant supervision and considerable assistance with her routine daily activities, and this assistance could be procured from a number of local home health agencies. Grace helped me select an agency that seemed to offer a desirable level of care.

Maria bade an emotional farewell to the caring staff that had assisted her through the past ninety days. She had written them a message depicting herself as Alice wandering through the unknown territory of Oz, and some members of the staff were depicted as helpers in this terrifying journey. Grace and Mary greeted Maria at the house as I pushed her in the wheelchair up the new ramp. Rosie was beside herself when Maria came into the house. Welcome signs and balloons added to the momentous occasion. A home health aide arrived within a few minutes. Maria was home at last after almost four months of unrelenting assaults to her being.

The home health aide was a complete disaster. The assistance that she gave Maria was minimal, and she sat watching TV for most of the four days that she was there. Before the next aide from the agency came out, Maria fell from the side of the bed while trying to get up by herself. Paramedics from a nearby fire station were called. They lifted her back in bed after determining that she was OK. After a called conference in Dr. Gates's office, Maria was readmitted to the skilled nursing facility, but she was in the area where chronic patients were housed. She left the small room that she shared with another bedfast patient three times each day for meals in the dining room. I visited her each day and took her for walks in the hall around the facility or took her for rides in the wheelchair to the lobby of the facility. We were both so very depressed during the ten days that she endured the miserable stay.

Mary helped me find a very reliable home health licensed practical nurse that agreed to come live in the house and take care of Maria for four weeks. Maria blossomed with the attention and care that she received. A physical therapist and an occupational therapist were sent by an agency to provide therapy three times each week for four weeks. Maria's progress was spectacular. The physical therapist had her walking up and down stairs, down the long driveway and back, and around the front yard walkway with assistance. Maria was almost able to dress herself with supervision and minimal assistance by the time the occupational therapist completed her assigned duties. The evening before the very capable home health nurse left, we had a celebration party of thanks to her and our many friends who had made it possible for Maria to be functioning at this level back in her own home.

Arrangements were made for Maria to receive physical therapy at a nearby outpatient facility. I drove her to the facility twice a week for the next six weeks. Her balance and muscle strength improved considerably. Home health aides were employed to stay from 11:00 p.m. to 8:00 a.m. seven days per week, and others came from 11:00 a.m. to 6:00 p.m. five days per week to assist Maria with routine activities, ambulating, and general care. She continued to walk around the front yard with assistance, and she enjoyed being out in the open spring air. Rosie was her constant companion on these walks. Life seemed to be settling into a busy but predictable routine, even though there was an almost constant stream of strangers in and out of the house to assist with Maria's care. She was doing so well that I planned a trip to visit my niece and her family in Fort Worth for four days, the last few days in April. We made arrangements for Maria's niece, Tammy, to stay with Maria during this much-needed respite.

We returned from physical therapy late one afternoon. Maria was in the wheelchair in the living room, and I had decided to take a short nap. I was awakened by her calls of, "Help! Help!" I found her in the kitchen next to the sink. She had fallen while trying to get a drink of water. She told me that her left leg had just folded under her. The paramedics came immediately, and after their usual thorough examination, an ambulance was called to take her to the emergency room. After determining that she was having cardiac arrhythmias and that her blood pressure was excessively high, she was admitted to the hospital. She would be seen by her cardiologist the following day. I canceled the home health aides and returned to my almost empty house and back to square one.

Her cardiologist implanted a cardiac pacemaker the evening before Tammy was to arrive. Maria went through the procedure well, and plans were made for her to come home in forty-eight hours. After Tammy arrived on the shuttle from the airport, I took her immediately to the hospital to see her aunt. After some discussion, we decided that I should go ahead with my planned visit the following day to Fort Worth.

I went by to see Maria before I left, and I told her that I would call her often. She assured me that she would be just fine with Tammy. She was to be discharged that afternoon, and one of the home health aides would be coming for eight hours on each of the days that I was gone. I left reluctantly for the airport shuttle.

It was sheer luxury to be waited on by my niece, Denise, and Josh, her husband. After four days, I felt almost human again. We went to a play one evening; we went out to eat several times; and we just relaxed, watched TV, and talked. I called Maria after she had gotten home from the hospital. She and Tammy were doing fine, even though she was a little weak. The home health aide had been there soon after Maria arrived home, and she had walked around the house with the aide a couple of times.

When I called on Sunday morning, Tammy answered the cell phone. She told me that they were back in the hospital. Maria had developed a severe case of diarrhea the day before and was so weak that she could hardly get out of bed. The home health aide had stayed with them until late in the evening and had advised that Maria be taken by ambulance to the emergency room early the next morning. Maria had not been able to keep any food in her stomach for the past twenty-four hours. She was very dehydrated and was receiving massive doses of intravenous antibiotics. We agreed that there was nothing I could do, so I would wait until the next day to return home as planned. The festive dinner that Denise had planned as a prebirthday celebration kept me from worrying about Maria.

I arrived as scheduled at the airport shuttle station, and Tammy and I went immediately to see Maria in the hospital. She was very pale and could hardly extend her hand to greet me when I came to her bedside. Dr. Gates had told her that she had picked up a very virulent bug when she was in the hospital the previous week for the insertion of the pacemaker. The necessary ninety days that Medicare required had transpired, and she would be going back to the skilled side of the previous skilled nursing facility when her present condition warranted her discharge. The positive effects of my brief respite were soon diminished.

I took Tammy to the airport shuttle the next day and thanked her profusely for being and staying there when she was so sorely needed. She and Maria had spent considerable time saying their tearful good-byes. I think that Tammy realized she might never see her aunt alive again.

There had been an almost complete change of personnel at the skilled nursing facility. The routine became much the same, but Maria was so weak that she could not participate fully in the expected activities. Her appetite was poor. She started skipping meals. She was obviously depressed. She was having a brownish discharge from around her vagina and rectum. The social worker called me in for a consultation visit and asked that I try to get Maria to become more involved in her therapies. When I talked with Maria, she said that she would try. "The food is tasteless. The therapists are pushy, and the aides are not very friendly. I am so miserable. I just want to go home."

I dealt with the mounting paperwork required for numerous agencies that had been involved with her care for the past nine months. I processed all of the papers necessary for becoming her power of attorney and filed them with each of the agencies that required this legalese. It seemed to be a never-ending process in which additional information was required immediately. My visits with Maria were quite depressing, but I tried to cheer her up and to keep her informed about what was transpiring at home and with her business affairs. She responded halfheartedly. She had very few visits from our previously supportive friends.

After four weeks at the skilled nursing facility, the social worker told me that there would be a conference the following week that I should plan to attend. At the conference, the therapists reported that Maria was not motivated to participate during her therapies. The nurse said that she had been skipping more meals and did not drink water. In short, she would be discharged within a week, and I should start looking for an assisted-living facility for her continued care. I was unbelievably stunned.

The social worker gave me the names of "the better" assisted-living facilities in the area. I apprised Grace of the new dilemma. She received an e-mail list of five facilities that had top ratings from the state health department. After visiting one of the facilities, I contacted Dr. Gates. He informed me that personnel in that facility had violated several of his medical directives, and he no longer took care of patients there. I visited two other facilities, but Grace and I crossed them off because of reported personnel problems. The fourth facility was just a mile away from the house. I asked the director many questions, and then Grace came over and asked still further questions. All seemed well except that they only had semiprivate rooms. The director met with Maria, the social worker, and me at the skilled nursing facility, and we decided to take the room. I could not give a definite date that Maria would be admitted, but I would know by the following Monday.

In the meantime, Grace had checked out the fifth facility on her list and reported that it was very clean, well kept, and in a nice area of private houses. The man that was in charge seemed a bit gruff and grumpy, but otherwise he answered all of her questions. I stopped by to meet the man, and I told him I was just looking. All seemed to be as Grace had reported.

I called the director of the place that we had decided on and said that we would be there on Friday morning. She abruptly told me that she had already filled the one vacancy, and she did not foresee others in the near future. My language following the brief phone conversation was quite profane. I called the social worker early the next morning and told her of the radical change of plans, and she was absolutely floored that there was someone so uncaring in the community. I immediately contacted the man at the last facility that we had visited and asked if Maria and I could come out for an interview and inspection of the facilities. We went out that afternoon. Indeed, Stephen, the owner and primary caregiver of the facility, seemed to be rather severe in our initial exchanges, but as we met his wife, Helen, and their five-year-old son, Anthony, it became evident that they were very caring people. The facility was incredibly clean and tidy. The private room into which Maria would be moving was bright and cheerful, with a three-quarter bed, a dresser, a large TV, a bedside stand, and a colorfully decorated stuffed chair. It looked like a well-decorated bedroom in any of the surrounding private homes.

I asked Stephen about the infraction that had been reported at the last health departmental visit having to do with medications. He explained that he had been using an outdated drug formulary but had a revised one now. After further discussion, we agreed that Maria would be moving in on June 15, 2012, at 10:00 a.m. What a relief! Maria and I were so grateful to Grace for all of her superb assistance. She had actually found the place, and it seemed to be the right one.

The move in was uneventful. Maria was so weak that she stayed in a wheelchair. Stephen gently assisted her out of the car and into her new bedroom. Lunch would be served at noon. He showed her the bathroom and told her to use the little bell attached to her bedside rail when she need help. Helen told me that Maria would only need three changes of clothes; Helen did the laundry twice a week after a shower. I picked up the new order of medications from the nearby pharmacy and gave Dr. Gates an update on Maria's welfare. He would see her in his office early the next week.

Maria's condition had deteriorated considerably during the last stay at the skilled nursing facility. She weighed

117 pounds compared to 150 at the time of her stroke less than one year earlier. She was able to take only a few steps, and she required extensive, constant assistance. Her pronunciation was much less distinct. She rarely smiled, and she lay in a fetal position in her new bed. Stephen took her to the dining table in a wheelchair, and Maria was placed at the head of the table. After brief introductions to the other four patients, Maria took a few bites and then asked to be excused. Back in her room, she started crying and kept saying over and over, "I want to go home. I want to go home." I tried to calm her down by saying that we should give the place a try for a few weeks. She finally drifted off to sleep.

At the appointment in his office, Dr. Gates told us that we needed to get hospice services started right away because Maria had "failure to thrive syndrome." We were both aghast at this sudden, unexpected pronouncement, and we left the office in tears. I drove Maria over to the house and brought Rosie out to see her where she sat in the car. Rosie was her usual exuberant self and seemed to be upset when I put her back in the house. Maria told me that she did not want to have hospice services because she was not ready to die. Again, I asked her to give it a try for a couple of weeks, and I said that I would be there with her all the way.

Dr. Gates had told me that the brown discharge from Maria's bottom was from a fistula that had formed between the rectum and vagina, and it may have extended into the bladder. The fistula had formed following a massive infection that she contracted in the hospital following her heart pacemaker implant. Usually, massive doses of antibiotics were given intravenously in such conditions, but her veins had collapsed to such an extent that they could not be used. She received several intramuscular antibiotic injections during the next few days.

I automatically tightened my protective armor of resolve to ward off the unabated penetrations of doom and despair that were overwhelmingly consuming my being and my soul. Emotions had to be set aside to face the reality that Maria's condition was deteriorating and the likelihood of her returning home without full-time assistance was almost nil. Tears and expressions of anguish and sorrow must be dealt with in the darkness of solitude. Moreover, the show at home must go on. The pets needed daily attention, meals had to be prepared, laundry had to be done, bills had to be paid, and the house had to be kept clean and in order. Thank goodness for the frequent e-mails regarding Maria's health status from Grace to friends and family that kept the phone calls under control. Life was bearable, but barely. I knew that I was becoming increasingly depressed, but I could not develop a plan of action to try to deal with it. It was always the bitter reality of unwavering circumstances that greeted me in the morning after mostly sleepless nights. I took comfort in Honey and Rosie, even though their demands always took priority over my needs.

The nurse, home health aides, and physical therapist from hospice services were graciously compassionate with Maria. They assisted her with bathing, dressing, and ambulating with a cane. She started eating her meals and conversing with some of the other residents at the dining-room table. She immediately became fond of Anthony and enjoyed his display, each evening at dinner, of the arts and crafts that he had completed.

I brought a medium-sized TV from home that gave better reception than the old one in her room, so that she could enjoy her favorite programs. Grace installed an audiovisual set so that Maria could watch movies, but she never learned how to operate the machine. She started reading the daily local newspaper and initiated conversations about current events. Her pronunciation of words returned slowly. She began using her cell phone to call her family and friends. Even though she had frequent bladder infections (probably from the fistula) and had to receive massive doses of intramuscular and oral antibiotics, and later continuous probiotics, Maria's condition resumed its previous course of improvement following her move to Reed's Road. After sixty days with the hospice-care personnel, Dr. Gates decided that their services could be discontinued.

As a celebration of her improving condition, Maria asked me if I would make arrangements to spend a few days in Sedona, a nearby resort in which we had spent so many luxuriously restful and exceedingly happy days.

After getting Dr. Gates's OK, I booked a two-bedroom cabin along the river for three days. A friend went with us to assist with Maria's care. The back of the RV was filled with all the paraphernalia that Maria had requested, along with the wheelchair, walker, and bedside commode that were her constant companions. There was little room for my clothes or for the food that we took for the short trek.

The rippling sound of the water splashing over the river rocks was tranquilizing. The tall pine trees and the overhanging mountain rocks added to the tranquility of this isolated garden of Eden. Maria seemed mesmerized by the sound of the rippling stream that was just outside the large glassed wall of the cabin. She ignored the several magazines that I had brought and decided that she would wait to go through the catalogs to order Christmas presents. Our friend and I helped her with toileting, bathing, and dressing. We went for a long drive up the canyon one day and ate lunch in a roadside restaurant. We spent the remainder of the brief time relaxing and enjoying the solitude of this pristine environment. Even though Maria required constant supervision and considerable assistance with daily self-care activities, the trip was declared a tremendous success. We could not have made the trip without our friend's help.

I met a new neighbor, Doris, who agreed to take Rosie for walks three times each week. I talked with Maria about selling her car, since it had been driven little during the past year. She said, "Absolutely not! I will be coming home in a few weeks, and I will need my car to go to the doctor." I told her that she could buy a new car when she got home, but she steadfastly refused to allow me to sell her car. I did not press the matter, and I continued to pay the insurance premium. I felt that confronting her with the reality of never driving again would not accomplish any real purpose.

I arranged with Caroline, a friend who was a home health aide, to pick Maria up from Reed's Road and bring her home for brunch each Sunday. I cooked foods that I knew Maria enjoyed, and she consumed the small portions and a small glass of wine with relish. After the meal, she sat in the special lifting recliner that I had bought her, and Rosie jumped up in her lap to be petted. Caroline assisted her to the bathroom and helped her wander through the house that had been so familiar to her just over a year ago.

Dr. Gates ordered six weeks of physical therapy on an outpatient basis at the rehab hospital. Caroline and I took turns taking her for the visits. Maria's ability to ambulate with assistance improved with their capable assistance. Maria came home for Thanksgiving, Christmas, her birthday, and New Year's with Caroline's help. She seemed to be thriving quite well with the care that she was receiving from Stephen and Helen at Reed's Road. Her numerous bladder infections slowed her down for several days about every three weeks. Strong antibiotics were ordered for ten days after each bout. This prolonged process entailed a visit to Dr. Gates's office, where the urine was sent away for a culture and a response from the laboratory specifying which antibiotic would be effective against the identified urinary organism.

Decision makers at Maria's long-term-care insurance office finally accepted the information that had been sent almost every week for nearly a year and started paying the statements that Stephen sent them each month. The cost of her care, including medications and transportation to various doctors, totaled over five thousand dollars each month. Most of this amount was covered by the several insurance policies that she had purchased and by Medicare. It became my responsibility as designated power of attorney to keep an accurate account of the numerous transactions in a timely manner.

I finally told Maria that I was selling her car and that she could buy a new one when she started driving again. She reluctantly agreed, and I was able to sell it within a couple of weeks to a healthcare friend. Someone told me that Maria cried for several days after the car was sold. I realized that it was still another blow to her fight for independence, but we did not talk about the matter.

The unrelenting stress that had consumed my life for the past eighteen months was taking a profound toll on my physical and emotional life—and my entire being. I was absolutely exhausted and inextricably drained. I had no life of my own. Was being a caregiver to be my role for the remainder of my life? Frankly, I did not feel the desire to prolong my life in such a miserable state. Yet, I felt an unwavering responsibility for Maria and for Rosie and Honey. There was no one to step in to help me with my endless burdens. I was trapped in a corner. I needed assistance to get out of this imprisoning corner, but I did not know where to turn. Feelings of entrapment extinguished my essence.

Five

Escape to Reality – Juanita Murphy

The actual experience of providing assistive health-care to a loved one over a prolonged period is both arduous and demanding. The caregiver role is decidedly different from what one might have observed as others enacted the role. I observed my mother providing for care for my disabled, blind dad for over twenty-two years. She and my brothers took care of a large farm and ranch with a large herd of cattle for fifteen years after my father became blind. She sold the farm/ranch to my older brother, and she and Dad moved into the small town near where they had lived for about thirty years. Dad moved about the house with a wooden cane, and he rarely left their home. He sat in a rocking chair in the living room from early morning until late evening and listened to the radio. The volume of the radio was always high because of his hearing loss. Conversations were difficult and loud. Until the last few years of his life, he walked to the kitchen table for his meals that Mother had prepared, walked to the bathroom, and then to bed at night. After a couple of falls, he was bedfast. Family and friends helped, but the burden of Dad's care fell on my mother's shoulders for twenty-two years, day after day. There were no other facilities available to care for him. Besides, she was expected to take care of her husband. The same expectation remains today.

As a nursing professor, I learned a great deal about the role of spousal caregiving from my graduate students who conducted research regarding ramifications of prolonged caregiving. We derived two significant findings from this research. First, spousal caregivers often died before their disabled spouses, even though they were in relatively good health at the outset of caregiving. Second, loss of social support was highly correlated with a spousal caregiver's failing health, and to life-threatening situations, and again to unexpected early death. The findings from these and numerous other nationally based research projects led health practitioners to the conclusion that caregivers need to develop new coping strategies, particularly if the care recipient's disability is prolonged. New services for elderly caregivers, such as respite and transportation assistance, have been implemented. However, these important research projects did not prepare me for the demands that were an integral part of the actual care-giving experience I encountered with Maria.

What had I learned from my mother's prolonged caregiving experience and from the numerous spousal caregivers who had been involved in the research projects? Foremost, I learned that it is imperative for caregivers to take care of their own health. If caregivers are to meet the needs of their loved ones, they must remain as healthy as possible, or they, too, will succumb to illnesses and disabilities. The realization that my own health was in jeopardy provided the impetus for me to slowly develop a perspective that assisted me in escaping from the enveloping trap of anger, depression, and resentment about my life in general. I knew that my physical, emotional, and mental health had deteriorated during the past two years.

A general assessment of my physical health made me aware that I rarely ambulated outside the house. Continuous acute back pain limited most of the activities that I had enjoyed previously. My friend Angie suggested that I contact a massage therapist who she had used. I followed her suggestion and was walking for short distances without a cane after two months of weekly therapy. The severity of my back pain abated somewhat so that I no longer used the TENS (transcutaneous electrical nerve stimulation machine), a pain-relieving apparatus that I had purchased. I began exercising twice weekly at a nearby therapy center to increase muscular strength and flexibility, and I continued massage therapy on a monthly basis.

Progress toward a projected goal of increased ambulation with decreased pain was slow and often disheartening. When lack of progress seemed overwhelming, I thought of my mother and realized the anguish and pain that she had endured as a caregiver. I recalled the numerous subjects in our research projects and the thousands of caregivers who feel pain, frustration, and depression just as I did. How were they dealing with the numerous challenges on a daily basis? It occurred to me that most of them never gave up. I thought, "If they can do it, I can do it." I felt a real sense of interconnectedness with those who were and are devoted caregivers. With the increased life expectancy and the resultant rapid aging of our society, I realized that our numbers are increasing daily. I tried to think through palatable solutions to a growing societal problem. These thoughts and questions gave me some insights regarding the accommodations I needed to make to escape my feelings of entrapment and return to the real world outside myself.

A friend informed me of a newly formed community program that was designed to help seniors, caregivers, and senior-service agencies with information about available services and support groups. I found that one of the most assistive facets of the Senior Connections was a weekly informational presentation on topics such as caregiver burnout, need for regular exercise, securing long-term-care insurance, employing a fiduciary to manage your finances, developing a will or trust, and when and where to secure needed services and meeting the challenges of aging. The participants in these sessions were facing many of the same challenges and problems that I faced daily. We each were seeking some escape from our overwhelming burdens.

Increasingly, I realized that I had to face the reality of the situation so that I could develop strategies to cope with the immeasurable stress. As I began to peel away the encumbering layers of the situation, I concluded that I had choices regarding the restraints that seemed to be controlling my life. I began to enumerate what I perceived to be issues and situations that were best managed by others and then selected out those that I should and could continue to manage.

The reality was that Maria's level of recovery from the stroke was much better than had been initially projected. She had endured and benefited from the various therapies she had received. However, she would need continued assistance and supervision with routine self-care activities and ambulation indefinitely for twenty-four hours each day and every day of the week. We had tried to secure services to provide this level of care in the home, and it had been a dismal failure for both Maria and me. It seemed obvious to almost everyone that she was receiving good care at Reed's Road and seemed to be content there. Her social interactions with the outside world with former friends had diminished. I encouraged her to call family members and friends. I concluded that she did not need to rely on me for her everyday physical care. I felt that my energy could best be focused on her business and financial affairs related to her estate and the daily management of her healthcare expenses. As her power of attorney, I made it a point to keep her informed about and involved in decisions regarding all of these activities. I valued her input, since she knew more of the intricate details of her estate than I did.

Additionally, I decided that I could spend less time with Maria at Reed's Road and that I should concentrate on the quality of the time we spent together. We went to the movies almost weekly and ate out a few times each month. Lifting the wheelchair out of the back of the car was an enormous problem for me. However, Maria was unable to walk the distance into the theater or restaurant, so the wheelchair was necessary. Even more difficult for me was assisting her out of the wheelchair and back into the car. After each trip, I would have acute lower back pain for two or three days. However, I did it with concentrated effort because these outings were important to both of us. She came home for Sunday brunch and to see Honey, the cat, and Rosie, the dog, almost every week. I paid a friend to help move her around the house in a wheelchair. Maria called me several times each day. She related what she had eaten at each meal and discussed her activities, plans, needs, and general welfare.

She read the local newspaper and told me what was happening in the community. She gave me critiques of the movies that she watched on the classic-movie channel. She told me about her encounters with other patients at Reed's Road and about her numerous conversations with little Andrew.

My move from desperation and depression to a more positive and realistic outlook on life was not a straight line, but a wavering configuration of difficulties as new obstacles arose. Maria's frequent bouts with bladder infection needed my constant monitoring, and they usually entailed an office visit with Dr. Gates every two or three weeks. New medications were ordered after each of these episodes, and I picked the medications up at the pharmacy and took them to her. I was astounded that she knew the side effects as well as the projected purpose of each medication that she received.

After more than a year of attempting to live a healthier lifestyle and to face reality with a greater sense of confidence, I began to feel that I had accomplished my goal to a small degree of success. I started channeling my energies into recovering friends that I had likely driven away in my prolonged state of depression. This was quite difficult, since many of our previous friends had moved into their own encounters with life's struggles. Some faced deteriorating health, and others were looking for new experiences in life.

My extrication process from "gloom and doom" included an irresistible impulse to travel and to leave my mountain of responsibilities behind. Could I do it? I decided to go for it, and I made arrangements to fly to Seattle to visit a great niece and her husband. I had unsettling trepidations about my abilities to get to the Phoenix airport, go through the airport, board the plane, and then participate in the various activities that Elaine and Mack had planned. However, I arranged for a wheelchair to transport me through the airports, and I found that going through security in the wheelchair was a breeze. I kept my fold-up cane with me to validate my disabilities. After all my worries, I had no problems going to Seattle or returning home.

We had an enjoyable three days on the beaches and touring the base where Mack was assigned. It was just great to sit around and talk about life in general. I called Maria twice a day, and she assured me that she was doing fine. The time away from my stressful situation and the revitalizing fun with Elaine and Mack restored my being, and I became more confident that I could start making plans for my unpredictable future. The next few days after the trip added to the emerging confidence that I should expedite the planning process.

The day after I arrived home, however, I received a call from a neighbor to tell me that there was an immense brush fire on the other side of the nearby mountain range and that it was traveling rapidly in our direction.

I could see the black smoke in the distance. He assured me that the fire was on the other side of the mountains and that it would never clear the top of the mountain. He added that firefighters were already on the scene and we were safe.

I had not seen Maria since my return, so without worry, I went over to Reed's Road to visit her, and then I stopped by the grocery store on my return trip home. As I approached the street to turn off to our house, I could see the brilliant orange flames spiraling up toward the sky and the dense black smoke that was moving along rapidly with the wind. There were innumerable cars parked along the streets, and crowds of people were outside their cars, viewing the terrifying holocaust that had moved down the side of the mountains toward my neighborhood.

I began to panic as I called my neighbor, Doris, and her husband. She told me to gather my valuables, some clothes, the pets and their food, and put everything in the back of my car. She said that we should be ready to evacuate in fifteen minutes. The phone rang just as I finished filling the back of the car with all the items that I had collected. My friends, Dot and Sue, told me to have all of my stuff together and in the car because they were coming by in five minutes to evacuate the pets and me. Dot added that the pets and I would be spending the night at their house that was some distance away from the fire. I called Doris to let her know of my change in plans.

When Dot and Sue arrived, they added several items to those that filled the back of my car. I put the pets in Dot and Sue's car and then drove my car to their house.

The hasty evacuation had happened so quickly that I was unable to comprehend the possible devastation that was eminently approaching from the encroaching flames. We learned from continuous news reports that the wind had blown the fire away from my neighborhood, but as the fire moved in a different direction, a sizeable number of people had been evacuated. Many of them were friends who lived less than a mile from our home. Fortunately, there was very little property damage.

After a sleepless night with Dot and Sue, the pets and I returned home. The charred side of the mountains attested to the magnitude of the fiery holocaust. I was the only person in my immediate vicinity that had evacuated. I was so thankful that everything was intact in the house and yard. I was numb with fear for several days as I realized that only a sudden change in the direction of the wind had kept the house and all its contents from becoming a large pile of smoldering ashes.

This frightening episode provided another turning point for me as I continued to map out my plans. This gorgeous log house and the large, park-like yard had been home to Maria for almost twenty years. However, since her stroke almost two years before, I had been encumbered with constant demands associated with maintaining the house and yard, which was six miles outside of town. Additionally, the upstairs portion of the house was rarely used, and the steep stairway could become a hazard. I felt that it was time to downsize.

I carefully approached Maria with the idea that I needed to move from this high-maintenance residence to a smaller house with a much smaller yard and closer into town. She seemed to agree and asked, "When?" I answered, "Soon." I learned that Maria had cried for days about this decision and repeatedly said, "I do not have a home anymore. Where will I live?"

I readily understood Maria's feeling about this home that she had adored for so long and the security and contentment that she had felt while living there. She had planned and orchestrated the interior decoration of the house as well as the landscaping on the large yard. She had selected the trees, plants, and bushes, and she carefully tended them after they were planted. She had an irrigation system installed that provided needed water to a raised vegetable garden, a large bulb garden, and several smaller flowerbeds, as well as the newly planted trees and plants. In short, she had been the author and the caretaker for this sizeable estate that was now going to be sold to some stranger.

Even though I sympathized with Maria's feeling about the house, and the stabilizing force that it was in her ever-changing world, I had to face the reality that if she could come home (which was doubtful), she would never be able to help maintain the large house and yard. It was a huge dilemma that taxed my integrity.

However, my resolve to purchase a smaller house closer to the downtown area and to sell the home that Maria loved so much was fueled by the renewed self-confidence that I had experienced during my visit with Elaine and Mack. I talked the decision over with my friends, Betty and Angie. They assured me that this was a wise, overdue decision. A realtor was employed, and the laborious process began for finding just the right house in a neighborhood that met all of the criteria that I had projected.

It took eight weeks of almost daily, desperate searching and endless weighing of pros and cons of numerous houses before the right one was selected. The house went on the market at 8:00 a.m., and I made an offer within an hour after exploring the inside and outside thoroughly. The deal was closed in thirty days. Was it possible that I was now the owner of a new house? I was overcome with exhaustion from the horrendous adventure, but I felt triumphant that I had taken a vital, huge step toward regaining control of my life. I sent out an e-mail message to friends and family describing the awesome view from the back patio of a nearby lake and mountains.

I could hardly contain my excitement as I drove Maria over to see the outside of the house. She expressed her feelings of approval, particularly when I told her of my plans to make some alterations for the pets. She agreed with my plans to have an enclosed iron fence built around the small area behind the house so that Rosie could go out to "potty." She thought that it was a good idea to have the back patio screened in so that Honey could be safe and still be outside. Both pets had enjoyed the outdoors in the other house very much, and I thought that these additions might assist in their adapting to their new environment.

Maria expressed some feelings of being overwhelmed by another sudden change in her life. I included her in planning for which furniture would be moved from the other house and where it might best be placed. She reluctantly conceded that all the furniture that had been in 2700 square feet of space in the log house would not fit in the 1660 square feet of space in the new house. But she insisted that all of her clothes and personal belongings be transferred to one of the two bedrooms in the new house. What else could I do? Against my better judgment, I gave in.

A lecture offered by Senior Connection on downsizing helped me to make a scheduled plan for the move. After choosing a local moving company, furniture, household goods, and personal belongings, as well as outdoor tools, were separated into "stay" or "go" groups. Items in the "go" group were either packed or labeled as to where they would be placed in the new house. I called Maria when I had questions about which items should go in each of the piles. She rarely said, "Stay." She wanted to retain everything.

A floor plan of the new house was drawn up, and sheets of paper were placed on the floor indicating where each piece of furniture would go. The new house was thoroughly cleaned, shelves were lined with new coverings, and some repair painting was completed. The move went smoothly, as did the estate sale that took place the following week. Not all of this could have been accomplished so expeditiously if Denise, my niece from Fort Worth, had not been there to help me for over a week. Also, several friends, including Betty and Angie, not only helped me with packing and unpacking, but also with problem solving when emergency contingencies arose, which was almost daily. I kept Maria apprised of the numerous everyday activities before and during the move. She usually had some suggestions regarding how and what should be done. Our lovely log home, in which we had spent several years of our lives, was put on the market.

Grab bars that had been in the vacated house were transferred to the new house. Furniture was arranged so that Maria could use either a wheelchair or walking cane to maneuver around the house. She often asked where she was going to sleep when she moved home, since the bedroom that contained her clothes had been converted into a study, and a futon had been procured for overnight guests. My consistent reply was, "We will handle the situation when the time comes." I knew it was unlikely that she would be able to return home.

The move was quite an adjustment for the pets. Honey, the cat, cried constantly from midnight until morning the first night that we were in the new home. After that first night, she explored each room and selected her sleeping places. She particularly enjoyed the screened-in patio that allowed her to communicate with the birds and rabbits in the back yard.

Rosie, the dog, was another story. She had been accustomed to a huge yard in which she could run and roam ad lib. Now she was confined to a postage-stamp-sized space. Doris came over and took her for long walks several times a week, and I took her for short walks every evening in the immediate neighborhood. She was a very strong beagle, and one evening when we went for a short walk in the neighborhood, she pulled me over, and I fell headlong into the street. There were no fractures, but my face was bleeding in several places from the fall. I knew that I needed to make changes for Rosie soon. I reluctantly put her up for adoption. She made a tremendous transition with her new parents at their two-acre estate, where she runs and sniffs the fresh air. Both Maria and I still miss her.

It was difficult to make these huge transitions alone. I talked by phone with Denise, my niece, and Doris, my former neighbor, several times a week. Both Denise and Doris helped me to face the crushing reality of the severity of Maria's disabilities and the limited prognosis for much further improvement. I came to realize that I could do little to change either the disabilities or their impact on her future welfare or life. As I settled into the new living environment, I began to ask myself further questions about what I could do differently so that I would have a more positive attitude in order to face the innumerable challenges that occurred almost daily. I realized that there were thousands of other individuals in entrapping situations worse than mine. Did they, too, feel miserable, angry, and enormous bitterness with their life's situation? How were they dealing with the numerous challenges that arose daily? Were most of them more accepting of whatever was put on their plates? What further accommodations did I need to make to escape my feelings of imprisonment and to return to the real world outside myself?

Unexpectedly, but almost miraculously, I was invited to attend a chronic-pain-management program sponsored by the county health department. The twelve individuals, who attended the six, three-hour workshop sessions, described their experiences with chronic pain and how it had altered their lives. My level of pain was much less than that reported by most of the other participants. Particularly informational for me were comments by fellow participants regarding how they dealt with the constant chronic pain. I was deeply chagrined to hear that the existing healthcare system had little to offer for the treatment of chronic pain. Several of the other participants were left with the insinuation that their pain was not a reality but a fiction of their imagination. I was relieved to hear that few of them had succumbed to taking narcotics, even though they were prescribed.

We were encouraged to develop a written plan of action for every day of the week to deal with our chronic pain. I planned to increase the time spent at the activity center to one hour, three times each week, and to attend a meditation class. Additionally, I planned to pace the time I was spending at the computer.

Of particular relevance for me was learning about the circular relationship between chronic pain and stress. Chronic pain can lead to anxiety, depression, fatigue, frustration, and anger. One's level of stress can be intensified at any point in the vicious cycle. I realized that this was what I had been dealing with for several years. However, pain to stress, and back to pain, had intensified with the caregiving functions that I had been performing for the past three years. By the end of the program, I felt as if I had emerged from a cocoon and concluded that I was no longer alone with the pain, depression, anger, and stress that had been consuming me for many months.

Meditation helped me to acknowledge my negative feelings of discomfort, anger, sadness, and depression. This acknowledgment has made me patently aware that suffering and joy are part of being human and that working through obstacles is fundamental to growth during life's journey. Additionally, I have become more aware that life is very brief and impermanent. I have come to realize that each day should be perceived as a precious present and should be lived to the fullest.

I am discovering that each time I am faced with an obstacle, I must rise from the onslaught and keep going, no matter how painful the ordeal. There are helpful individuals and services to assist in dealing with numerous traumatizing events. It is up to me to make a concerted effort to obtain information regarding the availability of assistive services and to use those that are beneficial. After all, I am responsible for the fulfillment of my life for as long as I am physically and mentally capable.

These are difficult lessons to be learned at any stage in life. It seems I have to relearn or at least revisit them every day. The incorporation of mindfulness, a process of being aware of and experiencing an event as it unfolds, requires continuous, conscious effort. I confess that I am not always successful, but I am trying.

My newly adopted coping strategies were severely tested during the thirteen months that it took to sell the house. According to informed reports, the housing market was good in the area, and because of the more rural location, the exquisite landscaping, and the artistic architecture of the house, I assumed it would sell rapidly. The constant maintenance and almost weekly services required my presence at the house several days each month. It became a suffocating heavy load that seemed endless. When a firm offer was finally made, I agreed, even though the price was much lower than we hoped to get. Maria agreed. Again, I was triumphant over arduous circumstances and had survived.

Soon after the sale of the house, it was my pleasure to host a sizeable surprise party for Maria's ninetieth birthday. Several of her many friends gathered for the momentous occasion, and most were surprised by how healthy she seemed. It is almost incomprehensible for me to fathom the depth of despair that she has felt and the numerous obstacles with which she has had to contend following the massive, acute stroke almost four years ago. I have had to make decisions that have left her feeling that I am abandoning her. However, she is aware that her safety, comfort, and well being have always been foremost in my deliberations, and her basic needs have not been compromised. Truly, Maria's life has been exemplary for many of us.

Yes, at times I am very lonely, and I miss sharing experiences with Maria. We rarely talk about the future, but we share the numerous activities in which we are involved during the day. Inevitably, our relationship has been altered during her long-term, disabling condition. I try not to cry while I am with her, and she rarely sheds tears in my presence. It seems as if we are trying to be strong for each other. Perhaps this is not facing the total reality of a difficult situation, but I am trying my best.

It has taken me so long to realize that life is such a superb miracle and that each moment of our existence is precious. Neither denial nor depression assists in escaping the inevitable traps or corners in which we find ourselves. When we become embedded in difficult situations that seem to be rampant with insurmountable problems, we each must face that reality with an open mind. This often requires moving outside ourselves and seeking the assistance of others. My escape from pain and depression into reality will always be incomplete, but I am inching forward. I am trying to relish each precious moment with reality and an open mind. "My past was the present. And my future will be my present. The present moment is the *only reality* I ever experience."

S. Johnson, *The Precious Present* (Garden City, New York: Doubleday & Company, Inc.).

Six

PTSD: A Circuitous Journey – Jeffrey Nuse

I have what is commonly known as posttraumatic stress disorder (PTSD). I am a veteran of the Vietnam War, and like many other veterans, my everyday life has been changed in significant ways. I have recurring memories, which are sometimes nightmares, and flashbacks that are so vivid that I feel like I am back in the war zone. I often feel angry, anxious, irritable, and out of control. I lose interest in things that I really care about, and I have trouble sleeping. I often have difficulty getting along with my spouse, friends, and other family members. To put it bluntly, my life seems to be out of whack, and I am trying constantly to make sense of where I have been and where I am going on this circuitous journey.

I realize that not all veterans of the various wars that our country has been engaged in have PTSD. I began to wonder if there was something in my background that might have made me more susceptible to this debilitating disorder. I would describe my childhood as average. I was raised in the 1950s, and lived in California with my mother and stepfather. I only met my biological father for about an hour when I was in my thirties, and I have few lasting impressions of him as a real person.

My mother was a large, good-looking woman from a strong German family.

She obviously hated my biological father, and she often told me what a rat he was. He had gotten her pregnant and then went off with another woman who was also pregnant. She immediately moved me and my sister, who was twelve years older than me, to California. I am eternally thankful that she taught me how to prepare food and generally take care of myself. She was overly protective of me, and very controlling. When I was about eight years old, she told me that she and my biological father had never married.

My stepfather was a big man, over six feet tall, and he weighed over two hundred pounds. He was not well educated. He taught me that aggressive behavior was the main key to survival. I recall his discussion about how to fight with other kids. He advised me, "If the other kid is bigger than you, get a stick, and that will make the fight even." He was the referee at my first fight, and the other kid was beating me badly. Finally, I got one good shot on him and knocked him down. After I had pummeled him really good, my dad picked me up and said, "I said fight fair."

He used aggressive behavior as the primary approach toward raising me. His idea of discipline was to send me to an old chestnut tree to cut switches, with which he would then beat me from head to toe. He did not allow me to cry. I remember wearing a long-sleeved shirt to school to cover up the black-and-blue marks on my arms, legs, and back. The beatings happened quite often, and he rarely gave a reason for their occurrence. My mother never interfered with these beatings. Undoubtedly, the trauma that I suffered during my formative years from this excessively abusive behavior has left a decided imprint on the remainder of my life. The impact that his abuse has had on the onset and my management of PTSD is probably mammoth.

When I was about nine years old, I drank one of my dad's beers. Even though the temperature outside was hot, I felt like the coolest kid in the country. During the years that I was in high school, I was drinking beer almost every day, and I would sometimes get drunk.

I left my grossly dysfunctional family and joined the navy when I was seventeen. The commander at boot camp was a fatherly type, and he invited new recruits who were homesick to come to his office, if we wanted to. I took him up on the offer and sat in his office and cried. He listened to my sob story about my dysfunctional home situation and about how miserable and out of control I felt. He asked if

I would like to beat up on his metal locker. I said, "Yeah," and beat on his steel locker with my fists for a few minutes. I allowed my pent-up emotions to rise from obscurity through this primitive form of aggressive behavior. I felt better after the session with the locker. But I began to drink a lot, and I was involved in fights almost daily.

One weekend when I was home on leave, I learned that my neighbor girlfriend was pregnant. We had been having sexual intercourse frequently for almost a year. My mother kept me informed about my son's birth, and she was involved in his early formative years.

After boot camp, I was stationed in Guam for over a year. I had become a mechanic, and I worked in the engine room of a ship. I received my general equivalency diploma (GED) during that time. Life was OK, but I felt I needed more action. I volunteered to go to the active war in Vietnam in 1966.

I was assigned to a special offshore reconnaissance unit that was something like the Seals. The main objective of our unit was to protect maritime shipping by monitoring enemy traffic. Every night we patrolled the numerous streams that led out into the ocean. My main responsibility, as a diesel mechanic, was to assure the proper functioning of the ship's engine so that the combat unit members had a safe place to leave and return when they went ashore.

There was an almost constant exchange of gunfire and rocket fire, particularly at night. We had been meticulously prepared in basic training to harness our killer instincts in order to survive. Frequently, I joined the combat unit, as needed, and engaged in active combat with the enemy when commanded to do so. When members of our combat unit were killed or seriously injured, it was my responsibility to bag the bodies and float them to a pier, where they were picked up by the military police.

Several members of my combat unit were killed during the nearly two years that I was in Vietnam. I was there when many drew their last breath. The captain of one of the skimmer craft boats was hit by a rocket that completely disemboweled him. I helped unload his body onto the pier so that he could be shipped home to his loved ones. These traumatic ordeals unequivocally changed my life during the six years that I was in the navy.

I came from a strong Christian background. What do you do when you are sent into combat? All of my military training had instilled in me the absolute notion that you kill or you will be killed. This tenant was more ingrained in my being than was the biblical commandment, "Thou shalt not kill." I was doing my duty by killing people who were enemies of my country.

I had mixed emotions as I returned to the country for which I had fought and for which many of my buddies had given their lives. As I walked through the San Francisco airport, a hand reached out and caught the sleeve of my uniform. I saw the blur of a face that was starting to spit on me. My reaction was so fast that I doubt the spit had reached me before my fist reached his chin. I was not prepared for this kind of behavior, even though we had been briefed about the demonstrations against the Vietnam War and the returning warriors. Is this what I fought for? This question remains with me over forty years later.

I was twenty-three when I was discharged from the navy. I had no idea what I would do with the rest of my life. After arriving back in California, my stepbrother asked me to move in with him and his wife and three-year-old son, Matthew. I shared a bedroom with Matthew, and we became the best of friends. Matthew was my constant companion, and life started to make a little sense. I played with him in the evenings, after my stepbrother and I returned from a day's work as roofers. My biological son and his mother lived nearby, and I had my six-year-old son over frequently. He and Matthew particularly enjoyed the pancakes that I made for them on Saturday mornings. My son had been told that I was his uncle. This was later clarified.

One morning Matthew did not get out of bed as I was leaving for work. He told me that his leg hurt really badly. His dad and mom took him to the hospital, and they had not yet returned when I came home from work. My stepbrother called me early the next morning and told me that Matthew had died from spinal meningitis.

Suddenly, my world crashed. At just three years old, my new best buddy was dead. How cruel! How unforgiving! Another buddy was dead. I just lost it. I was unable to return to work.

The next almost twenty years are a blur of nothingness. I wanted to stop thinking, so I drank almost constantly. I was very explosive and got into lots of fights. I tried to numb my feelings with speed, heroin, and barbiturates. I had several insignificant jobs. The jobs did not last long, because I was so undependable. I would get drunk and forget to go to work. I lost my car and many of my personal possessions. After a few years, I did not have a place to stay, and I ended up on the streets. Several times I was picked up and taken to jail. My previous friends and family would have nothing to do with me. I got married a couple of times, but the marriages never lasted long. I did not want an intimate relationship in which I might reveal my innermost thoughts. My second son was born from the second marriage.

Feelings of exhaustion and helplessness were overwhelming. I felt that I was at the end of the road, with nowhere to turn. I felt cold and naked, and I knew that I had reached the bottom. I felt inescapably entrapped, and I could not find a way to gain control of my life. I was miserable, and I wanted to strike out at someone or something that I could blame for my feelings of hate, anger, and depression.

Additionally, I started having horrible dreams in which I was walking through a gorge of body parts and bloody intestines. I never see any faces, but all of the people are dead. These dreams have continued through the years, and they occur several nights in succession for one or two weeks. I have no idea what triggers their occurrence, and I cannot predict when they are likely to occur. Perhaps the dreams are an aftermath of all the deaths that I encountered during the war.

Even with the devastating aftermaths of the horrible dreams and the almost total loss of my being and existence, I never contemplated suicide. It did not seem to be a viable escape from my overwhelming entrapment. But I realized that my increasing dependency on alcohol and drugs would soon lead to a premature death. I needed help!

One evening I fell to my knees and prayed desperately. In essence, I said, "God, I am getting old. I am going to need some help. I need a place where I can hang my hat, a place to call home. If you can help me, I would really appreciate it." I had no place to turn except divine intervention.

Fortunately, I made some friends who worked in a recovery facility in a nearby town in California. They had been sober for several years, and they secured a room for me in the facility. I eagerly learned the principles of recovery. Those principles have kept me on a steady course of sobriety for the past twenty-five years. After six months, I left the recovery facility with renewed confidence that I could turn my life around.

I rented a room from one of the people who worked in the recovery house. I had no money or credit. I did not have a car or a driver's license. I obtained a couple of small jobs and procured a little money so that I could pay the rent. I was very frugal, and I started saving about half of my earnings. I did not buy clothes unless it was necessary.

Slowly, and with pain-staking effort, my recovery started. Often, I refer to this period as the beginning of my life. Yes, I had somehow made it through a traumatic childhood. However, the years following my childhood were almost a complete blank. I was now a forty-year-old adult, and my life seemed to be just starting.

My prayers for a job were answered when I filed an application and was hired by the city as a member of the tree crew. I became acquainted with a group of traffic operators, and I volunteered to help with a project that they were doing for the city. After two years as a mainte-nance assistant with the traffic operations department, I became crew leader, and then I was promoted to a senior management position for the city.

My second son came to live with me shortly after I started working for the city. At twelve years old, he was already drinking fairly heavily and into street drugs. My few parenting skills were stretched to the limit on numer-ous occasions as I tried to reason with him about what he was doing with his life. We both knew that I was a poor example, but he had no other place to turn. He left after an arrest for drug possession. I felt like a complete failure as a parent.

I was fifty-three years old when I met and married Donna. She, too, worked for the city. She was divorced and had two sons. It seemed that we had a lot in common.

I had been in the senior management position for about five years when I was diagnosed with prostate cancer. I went through surgery and seven weeks of radiation without any complications. After a couple of months, I went back to work. However, my tolerance for the constant complaints at work irritated me, and I was always on edge. Donna and I decided that I could quit working after we determined that my accrued retirement benefits were quite lucrative.

We purchased a house along the Oregon coast that we both loved. We viewed it as our retirement home. Donna worked for two more years while I made numerous treks up to our new home and did some minor renovations and general improvement.

The onset of symptoms of PTSD was sudden. I was sitting in front of our big, beautiful home in Oregon smoking a cigar. I was watching the trees sway on the six-acre spread that we loved. All of a sudden, it was as if I fell off the edge of the planet. I felt like I had an emotional break from reality, and everything seemed to change after just a brief moment. I told Donna about what had happened, and she scheduled a doctor's appointment for me at the Veterans Administration hospital in Medford within a few days.

I also told Donna about another incident that had happened a few days earlier. One morning, I awakened at about 4:00 a.m., and it was still dark outside. I suddenly looked down at myself. I had a pistol in my belt and a rifle in my hand. I was standing on a hill, some distance from our property. I thought that I was on patrol. I had no recollection of leaving the house or walking to the place where I stood with the rifle and pistol, ready to shoot. It was unbelievably frightening as I thought, "What am I doing here?"

I related the nature of my assignment in Vietnam to various VA personnel. A doctor who had followed my case told me that he thought I was having posttraumatic stress disorder. I had never heard of such a disorder, and I immediately became angry, confused, and frustrated. Why was this happening to me? A psychiatrist confirmed this diagnosis after learning about the nature of my activities in the Vietnam War.

I started taking classes at the VA hospital with a psychologist who was considered an authority on PTSD. I had an episode during one of the classes in which I lost contact with reality. The psychologist helped me to return to reality by using my five senses. She explained that I should use the same process whenever I felt the sensations start to come on. At last, I had some tools with which to work.

One of the most important things that I learned from the psychologist was that my symptoms are a psychobiologic reaction to stress rather than a sign of weakness or a character flaw. She encouraged me to deal with my painful memories and feelings about an abusive childhood, the Vietnam War experiences, and the twenty years that I had lost after returning home. She explained that I would need both psychotherapy and pharmaco-therapy indefinitely.

It was difficult to leave the excellent services that she and her colleagues had provided when Donna and I decided to move to Prescott, Arizona. I felt an urgent need to get away from the darkness and wet climate of Oregon, which reminded me so much of Vietnam.

The move was more stressful than I had anticipated, and I became immobilized. We were grateful that my second son was living with us at the time. He took over for me and helped at both ends of the move. I felt like an observer. I did not know what to do, and I was not able to connect with what was happening. I was so frustrated, and I could not explain what was going on inside my head. Donna and I had several spats, but I felt completely out of control.

I have begun to realize that there is no cure for my PTSD, and I must deal with it and adapt to it. I have periods during which I can stay in the present. I have decided that if I dwell on the past, I am sad and depressed. If I start thinking about the future, I become anxious. I try to concentrate on the reality of the present; however, it takes a lot of vigilance.

I never know what to expect of myself behaviorally. I can go from hope to despair in a brief moment. Sometimes these emotional changes occur as the result of too many people around; at other times, it may be too much noise; and still other times, it is just too much hubbub. I attempt to overcome these feelings of despair and impending doom by talking with friends at Starbucks almost daily. I rarely complete tasks around the house because of lack of ability to concentrate. I am usually hypervigilant and prefer to have my back against the wall when I'm in a crowded room. My daily life seems to be a never-ending vicious circle of adjusting to depression, hopelessness, and inadequacies. Medications have given me the ability to be more stable when some of these feelings occur unexpectedly.

My present feelings of entrapment are similar to those that I endured following the twenty years of alcohol and drug abuse during which I sank to the depths of despair. However, I use the same guiding principles of Alcoholics Anonymous today that I used to escape the self-inflicted entrapment of twenty years ago. I am expected to be responsible for myself and to be ready to assist others. I feel some degree of satisfaction when the several individuals that I sponsor in AA tell me of their personal and positive life changes. Perhaps I am fulfilling some purpose on this planet.

I have accepted the reality that I have to cope with PTSD indefinitely and daily. The circuitous journey that has led me to face this reality has also assisted me with learning to take one day at a time and to try to live it to the fullest, no matter what the circumstances. I am learning that escape from entrapment is possible if I face each day openly and honestly. On some days, I am more successful than others.

29980254R00090

Made in the USA
Middletown, DE
08 March 2016